Long-Term Hemodialysis

Contributor:

Alfred P. Morgan, M.D.

*Assistant Professor of Surgery, Harvard Medical School;
Senior Associate in Surgery, Peter Bent Brigham Hospital
—Boston, Mass.*

Long-Term Hemodialysis

The Management of the Patient with Chronic Renal Failure

SECOND EDITION

Constantine L. Hampers, M.D.

*Assistant Clinical Professor of Medicine, Harvard Medical School;
Senior Associate in Medicine, Peter Bent Brigham Hospital
—Boston, Mass.*

Eugene Schupak, M.D.

*Clinical Associate Professor of Medicine, Mt. Sinai Medical School;
Consultant in Nephrology, City Hospital at Elmhurst
—New York, N.Y.*

Edmund G. Lowrie, M.D.

*Instructor in Medicine, Harvard Medical School;
Associate in Medicine, Peter Bent Brigham Hospital
—Boston, Mass.*

J. Michael Lazarus, M.D.

*Instructor in Medicine, Harvard Medical School;
Associate in Medicine, Peter Bent Brigham Hospital
—Boston, Mass.*

GRUNE & STRATTON
A subsidiary of Harcourt Brace Jovanovich, Publishers

New York and London

Library of Congress Cataloging in Publication Data

Hampers, Constantine L
  Long-term hemodialysis

  Includes bibliographical references.
    1. Artificial kidney. I. Title. ¡DNLM: 1.   Hemo-
dialysis. 2. Kidney, Artificial. 3. Kidney failure,
Chronic—Therapy. WJ300 H229L 1974¹ ˢ
RC901.7.A7H3 1974 617'.461 73-14883
ISBN 0-8089-0819-7

Long-Term Hemodialysis
SECOND EDITION
  1973 by Grune & Stratton, Inc.
First Edition 1967

  Grune & Stratton, Inc.
  111 Fifth Avenue
  New York, New York 10003

Library of Congress Catalog Card Number 73-14883
International Standard Book Number 0-8089-0819-7
Printed in the United States of America

To our patients and staff

Contents

Preface

There has been great progress in the field of hemodialysis since 1967 when the first edition of this book was published. The progress made has been primarily in the application of the technique of hemodialysis to a larger number of people. The success of the artificial kidney in maintaining the life of the patient with chronic renal failure in a useful and productive manner is now underlined by federal legislation. In late 1972, Congress enacted and the President signed an amendment to the Social Security Act (PL-92-603) which effectively provides financial support for the care of the vast majority of patients with renal failure in this country. Financial coverage for kidney failure as a "catastrophic illness" sets a precedent which may be followed by coverage for other diseases.

We have rewritten this book at this time because there will most assuredly be an expansion of dialysis facilities throughout the country. We felt it would be useful to summarize in an up-to-date fashion the current state of the art. As before, we have been careful to separate opinion from fact, while presenting those practice techniques which we feel might be useful to the unexperienced person entering the field.

Doctors Lowrie and Lazarus have joined Dr. Schupak and me in writing the text, since we felt that expanding the authorship would allow a more balanced presentation. We have attempted in this edition to go into greater scientific depth regarding various aspects of renal failure.

This book is directed to a number of groups with varying degrees of involvement in nephrology: to nephrologists untrained in dialysis; to physicians and surgeons who are not nephrologists, but who are

interested in chronic renal failure and dialysis; and finally, to profession-
als other than physicians who are or intend to be intimately involved
in dialysis. Since the needs and interests of each group may differ
in certain respects, we hope each will understand and tolerate our
shortcomings.

C. L. Hampers, M.D.

Acknowledgments

The authors acknowledge with gratitude the assistance of the Medical Service, under the direction of Dr. George W. Thorn, Professor Emeritus, Harvard Medical School, and of the Surgical Service (Dr. Francis D. Moore, Chief) of the Peter Bent Brigham Hospital, in obtaining some of the original observations reported herewith. We also gratefully acknowledge the support of the Department of Medicine at the City Hospital at Elmhurst, under the direction of Dr. Stanley Seckler. We would especially like to thank Dr. John P. Merrill under whose tutelage we all trained. We are grateful for support and contributions from Doctors G. L. Bailey, E. B. Hager, J. E. Murray, R. E. Wilson, C. B. Carpenter, M. Neff, R. Slifkin and A. Baez. In our own area, we thank the Fellows of the Cardiorenal Section of the Peter Bent Brigham Hospital; the members of the Renal Unit at Elmhurst; and the nursing and technician staff of the Dialysis Units at both hospitals. We are also greatly indebted to the superb staff at our out-of-hospital units—The Babcock Artificial Kidney Center and Bio-Medical Applications, Inc. (Queens, N.Y.). Mrs. Elizabeth Simpkins and Miss Ruth Canty performed invaluable services in helping us with the manuscript.

1

Clinical Engineering in Hemodialysis

A hemodialyzer is basically a membrane separation device that functions as a mass exchanger during clinical use. Theoretically, it transfers noxious substances from the blood into dialysate so that they may be discarded. As such, an artificial kidney may assume, in part, the excretory role of its biological counterpart. However, it is obvious that there is no way in which hemodialyzers in their present form can assume endocrine or metabolic functions of the normal human kidney, and palliation of the uremic syndrome by dialysis is therefore limited.

Hemodialysis is becoming a common procedure in the armamentarium of clinical therapy, and great strides in dialyzer design have been made in recent years. To properly manage his patient a physician must have a thorough knowledge of physiology, pharmacology, and medicine and must keep abreast of developments in these fields. Similarly, the dialysis physician should have a functional knowledge of the physical principles involved during the operation of a hemodialyzer. A familiarity with the basic engineering principles allows him to more accurately predict the results of therapy and to decide upon rational treatment protocols. In addition, he will be required to make some judgement regarding new devices offered for possible clinical use and to interpret manufacturers' specifications.

The engineering principles involved in the operation of a hemodialyzer have been described in the literature [1–5]. This chapter reviews the basic concepts required to understand the operation and

1

evaluation of a hemodialyzer. Physical principles will first be presented and illustrations using commercially available dialyzers as examples will follow. No effort has been made to catalog or compare devices in current clinical use. We have attempted to minimize the mathematical aspects of the presentation, but some mathematical manipulation is necessary in a discussion of this sort. Nonetheless, the basic concepts are relatively simple and a knowledge of algebra is the only prerequisite to an understanding of the arithmetic involved. Even without this knowledge, we hope the reader can procure some insight into the general phenomena that occur during the operation of an artificial kidney. Appendix A defines the symbols employed.

Dialyzer performance can be conveniently divided into several broad categories. The most important and complex may be termed solute removal or *mass transfer*. In general, this constitutes the basic aim of hemodialytic therapy. Three of the remaining categories overlap somewhat. *Fluid removal,* for instance, is obviously an important aim of hemodialysis, and the rate of removal is proportional to the operating pressures within the dialyzer. *Flow resistance,* to be defined later, determines the operating pressures required to achieve a given blood flow rate. The compliance of the blood compartment determines the amount by which the *internal blood volume* will expand in response to a given increase in pressure. The last consideration, *blood recovery,* is important because blood loss should be minimized in patients with renal failure. These topics—mass transfer, pressures and flows, fluid removal, dynamic blood volume, and blood recovery—will be discussed in turn.

MASS TRANSFER

Figure 1 illustrates the general scheme of a hemodialysis system.

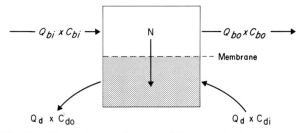

Fig. 1.   Flow scheme of a typical hemodialysis system. See Appendix for explanation of symbols.

The quantity of a solute such as urea entering the dialyzer in a given time is the product of the blood flow rate and solute concentration entering the dialyzer ($Q_{bi} \times C_{bi}$). By analogy, the amount of solute leaving the device may be estimated by the product ($Q_{bo} \times C_{bo}$). The flux or transfer rate across the dialyzing membrane into the dialyzing solution is clearly the difference between the amount entering and the amount leaving the blood compartment.

$$N = Q_{bi}C_{bi} - Q_{bo}C_{bo} \qquad (\#1)$$

Flux may also be estimated from dialysate flow and concentration. Figure 1 illustrates this point.

$$N = Q_{di}C_{di} - Q_{do}C_{do}$$

The rate of solute flux across the membrane is determined by the physical properties of the dialyzer and by the solute-concentration gradient across the membrane. Specific dialyzer properties of importance are the dialyzing surface area, the overall membrane permeability (or overall mass transfer coefficient), and membrane-sieving coefficient. Obviously, the permeability and the sieving coefficient of a given membrane will vary for different molecular species, being higher for small and lower for large molecules. The overall relationship may be described as follows:

$$N = (K_o \, A \, \Delta \bar{C}) + (s \, Q_f \, \bar{C}_b) \qquad (\#2)$$

This states that flux has two basic components—that due to diffusion (conductive mass transfer), which is represented by ($K_o \times A \times \Delta \bar{C}$), and that due to ultrafiltration (convective mass transfer), which is represented by ($s \times Q_f \times \bar{C}_b$). Convective transfer is the product of fluid filtration rate, blood solute concentration, and the sieving coefficient. The sieving coefficient is the ratio of blood solute concentration to filtrate solute concentration.

$$s = \frac{C_f}{C_b}$$

This expression and equation #2 represent a simplified concept of molecular sieving and define it as the fraction of molecules crossing the membrane with bulk fluid flow. Unfortunately, the relationship between conductive and convective transfer becomes very complex.

The solute concentration in the filtrand is greater than that in the filtrate, and this concentration difference promotes molecular movement by diffusion. Therefore, the ratio is really due to the combined effects of convective and conductive flows [6], and the coefficient as defined herein is not, strictly speaking, comparable to that defined by Pappenheimer [6]. Also, the sieving coefficient characteristically changes with changing Q_f, which further complicates the matter. Nonetheless, the relationship described in equation #2 serves to illustrate the general principles involved.

While urea and other solutes are removed by both convection and conduction in current clinical dialyzers, convection is a relatively minor source of waste removal except for one experimental prototype [7]. This is particularly true for relatively lower molecular weight species. As molecular weight increases, the relative importance of convective mass transfer increases. The molecular weight spectrum of uremic toxins is not known, however, and dialyzer performance is currently measured clinically by relatively small molecules such as urea and creatinine. Therefore, the remainder of our discussion will be limited to conductive or diffusive mass transfer, and equation #2 can be simplified to:

$$N = K_o A \, \Delta \, \bar{C} \qquad (\#3)$$

One can see from equation #3 that as surface area increases so does the capacity to remove wastes. Similarly, as permeability increases so does waste removal. Fick's law of diffusion [8] and equation #3 state that a third factor determining flux is the average blood-dialysate concentration gradient. As the gradient decreases so does the rate of solute removal. Hence, greater quantities of solutes are likely to be removed early in dialysis when the blood-dialysate solute concentration gradient is relatively high.

The concentration gradient here is a log mean gradient and can be estimated from the expression:

$$\Delta\bar{C} = \frac{\Delta C_{bi} - \Delta C_{bo}}{\ln(\Delta C_{bi}/\Delta C_{bo})} \qquad (\#4)$$

The blood-to-dialysate concentration gradients at blood inlet and outlet ports depend upon the flow geometry (relative directions of blood and dialysate flow) of the dialyzer. Four common geometries are used clinically. The two most common are countercurrent, in which blood and dialysate flow in opposite directions, and completely mixed, in which there is no measurable difference in dialysate solute concentration at any point on the membrane's surface. Cocurrent flow is relatively less efficient than countercurrent flow, and is not used clinically. The differences in blood and dialysate concentrations at blood inlet and outlet ports are referred to as boundary conditions and are illustrated in Table I for cocurrent, countercurrent, and completely mixed flow geometries. Crossflow dialysate distribution is relatively more difficult to evaluate mathematically and involves a summing of blood-dialysate concentration gradients at each point on the membrane. Graphs and tables for this type of analysis are available [9].

Table 1

Boundary Conditions for Various Dialysate-Blood Flow Patterns

Dialysate flow	ΔC_{bi}	ΔC_{bo}
Cocurrent	$C_{bi} - C_{di}$	$C_{bo} - C_{do}$
Countercurrent	$C_{bi} - C_{do}$	$C_{bo} - C_{di}$
Completely mixed	$C_{bi} - C_{d}$	$C_{bi} - C_{d}$

Further explanation of the overall mass transfer coefficient is in order. The reciprocal of permeability is resistance:

$$R_o = \frac{1}{K_o}$$

Overall mass transfer resistance in a hemodialyzer is composed of three separate components linked in series. The first of these is due to a blood film layer, the second is the resistance of the membrane itself, and the third is formed by a dialysate-fluid film layer:

$$R_o = R_b + R_m + R_d$$

Resistance, in turn, is determined by two film or membrane properties. It is directly proportional to the membrane thickness and inversely proportional to the diffusion coefficient of the molecule within the membrane or film—a measure of the ease with which a given solute passes through a given solvent.

$$R_o = \frac{t'_b}{D'_b} + \frac{t'_m}{D'_m} + \frac{t'_d}{D'_d}$$

Therefore, the thicker the membrane or fluid film, the greater will be the mass transfer resistance. The thickness of the dialysate fluid film may be reduced by increasing the velocity of dialysate flow over the membrane to promote turbulence. At relatively high flow rates the dialysate film resistance will be zero. Further, one original aim of the hollow fiber kidney was to reduce R_b by decreasing the thickness of the blood film barrier [3].

The rate of ultrafiltration in most commercially available dialyzers is very small compared to the total blood flow rate entering the device. Therefore, it is common clinical practice to assume the rates of blood flow entering and leaving the dialyzer are identical ($Q_{bi} = Q_b = Q_{bo}$) and very little error is introduced by making this assumption. Equation #1 can then be simplified to:

$$N = Q_b (C_{bi} - C_{bo}) \qquad (\#5)$$

If more precision is desired, a nontransferable substance such as protein or hemoglobin can be measured in the blood and Q_{bo} can be estimated.

$$Q_{bo} = Q_{bi} \frac{C_{bi}}{C_{bo}}$$

Unfortunately, the error involved in determining hemoglobin or protein concentrations is probably sufficiently great to offset the small error accompanying the assumption that inlet and outlet blood flow rates are the same under most clinical conditions.

The overall mass transfer coefficient can then be estimated by setting equations #3 and #5 equal to each other and solving for K_o:

$$K_o = \frac{Q_b}{A} \times \frac{\Delta C_{bi} - \Delta C_{bo}}{\Delta \bar{C}} \qquad (\#6)$$

The appropriate $\Delta \bar{C}$ can be estimated from equation #4 and the appropriate boundary conditions outlined in Table I.

Performance of hemodialyzers has traditionally been compared by clinicians through the use of the dialysance curve—a graph relating dialysance to blood flow rate. Dialysance is defined as the ratio of solute flux to blood-dialysate solute concentration gradient [2-5].

$$D = \frac{N}{C_{bi} - C_{di}} = \frac{Q_b(C_{bi} - C_{bo})}{C_{bi} - C_{di}} \qquad (\#7)$$

Dialysance is basically similar to clearance

$$Cl = \frac{N}{C_{bi}} = \frac{Q_b(C_{bi} - C_{bo})}{C_{bi}} \qquad (\#8)$$

except that the denominator for calculating dialysance is a gradient, and it will equal clearance if $C_{di} = 0$. The reason for using a gradient is clear from equation #3. As the concentration gradient decreases due to increasing dialysate concentration in a tank-type dialyzer, for instance, solute flux will decrease. Clearance will also decrease, even though the basic physical characteristics of the dialyzer have not changed. Therefore, dialysance, which is in part independent of gradient, has been used for comparing dialyzers.

Assuming a completely mixed or negligible dialysate solute concentration allows the simultaneous solution of equations #3, #4, and #5 to yield an expression for dialysance in terms of the pertinent system parameters, K_o and A.

$$D = Q_b \{1 - \exp[-(K_o A / Q_b)]\} \qquad (\#9)$$

This expression, often referred to as Rankin's equation [10], is useful for predicting the form of a dialysance curve from dialyzer specifications and demonstrates that the shape of this curve indeed depends on the dialyzer constants. Dialysance also depends on the rate of blood flow to the device, and clearance—as will be seen later (equation #10)—depends both blood and dialysate flow rates. The product, $K_o A$, is mathematically independent of both blood and dialysate flow rates and may be a more reliable parameter by which to compare dialyzer performance than dialysance. It is difficult to discern whether the shape of a dialysance curve is due to the normal dependence of dialysance on blood flow rate or some alteration in the basic operating constants of the device which accompanies changes in blood flow rate. Since $K_o A$ is independent of blood flow, any alteration in this product that is observed with changes in blood flow is likely due to some change in the system parameters of permeability or area.

Figure 2 illustrates the dependence of dialysance on blood flow rate. Dialysance increases rapidly at low flows and tends to level off at higher blood flow rates. The left side of the figure illustrates a dialysance curve for a theoretical device with a dialyzing surface of 1 square meter and an overall permeability of 3.33×10^{-2} cm/min. $K_o A$ is assumed to be constant, and the mathematical independence of this product on blood flow rate is illustrated. The right-hand portion of

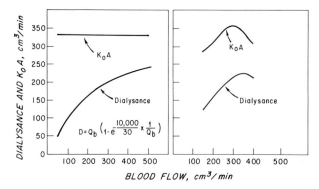

Fig. 2. Typical dialysance curves with the K_oA product also shown. Curve on the left is for a 1-square meter device with an overall mass transfer resistance of 30 min/cm for solute in question. K_oA does not change. Curve on the right represents device in which K_oA changes with changing blood flow rate. This also represents 1-square meter and the minimum resistance is 30 min/cm.

the figure illustrates a dialysance curve in which K_oA initially rises with increasing blood flow, reaches a nadir, and then decreases. The increasing K_oA with increasing blood flow could be due, for instance, to poor blood perfusion patterns at low flow rates and more favorable perfusion patterns at higher blood flow rates. With increasing transmembrane pressures that necessarily accompany higher blood flow rates, a greater fraction of the membrane may touch the supporting structures of the device resulting in loss of effective dializing surface area.

If one is primarily concerned with the performance of a device under a variety of operating conditions, K_oA is probably the relevant parameter by which hemodializers should be compared. If, on the other hand, one is concerned with patient effects, clearance is probably the relevant parameter, as will be seen later. However, the discussion is somewhat academic, since clearance can be estimated from K_oA, Q_b, and Q_d (e.g., equation #10).

Some discussion of the role of varying molecular weights on mass transfer and blood clearance is in order. By using the same logic employed in deriving equation #9, expressions for clearance can be derived. The precise expression clearly depends on the boundary conditions of the dialyzer. If, for example, one assumes a completely mixed dialysate delivery with a given fresh dialysate feed—used dialysate bleed rate (Q_d) such as is commonly employed with some coil systems (recirculating single pass) and steady-state conditions, equation #10 for clearance can be derived:

$$Cl = Q_b \frac{1 - \exp[-(K_oA/Q_b)]}{1 + Q_b/Q_d\{1 - \exp[-(K_oA/Q_b)]\}} \qquad (\#10)$$

This is a formidable-looking expression, but an understanding of its derivation is not necessary to see that clearance, like dialysance, is determined by the K_oA product and blood flow rate. The dialysate bleed-feed rate is also a determinent. K_oA represents the intrinsic mass transfer properties of the dialyzer and thus clearly contributes to its ability to transfer solutes. Decreasing blood flow results in decreasing dialyzer clearance, particularly when the ability of the dialyzer to transfer solute (K_oA) is high (e.g., for lower molecular weight solutes). This reduction in clearance at lower blood flow rates is caused by depletion of the substance in blood as it traverses the dialyzer, resulting in a reduction of the concentration driving force. The same general observation applies to reduced dialysate flow rates. As dialysate flow decreases, more time is allowed for blood and dialysate to reach a concentration equilibrium. As blood and dialysate concentrations approach one another, the concentration driving force is again reduced, solute flux (N) diminishes, and clearance falls. With increasing molecular weight, K_oA is smaller, the capacity of the dialyzer to remove solutes is less, and, within limits, the effects of altering blood and dialysate flow rates are diminished. The major relationships involve the relative capacities of (a) the blood to deliver solute to the membrane, (b) the dialysate to sweep it away, and (c) the membrane to transfer it. Any one of these factors can serve to limit total mass transfer.

If the quotient K_oA/Q_b is equal to or less than 0.1, the expression $\{1 - \exp[-(K_oA/Q_b)]\}$ may be approximated by K_oA/Q_b, due to the mathematical properties of exponents of e. To meet this condition at a blood flow rate of 300 ml/min, for example, K_oA should not exceed 30 ml/min. For a 1-square meter device, then, K_o should not exceed 3×10^{-3} cm/min (R_o = 333 min/cm). As molecular size increases, the mass transfer coefficient decreases and this decrease is marked for substances with molecular weights over 1000 for membranes in current clinical use [11]. The mass transfer coefficient for urea (molecular weight = 60) for a commonly used dialyzer providing 1 square meter of surface area is approximately 33.3×10^{-3} cm/min (K_oA = 333 ml/min), while for substances of molecular weight slightly over 1000 this value is in the range of 1.66×10^{-3} cm/min (K_oA = 16.6 ml/min). It is clear then that K_oA will become smaller with increasing molecular weight.

For substances of sufficiently large molecular weight such that K_oA/Q_b is less than 0.1, equation #10 then reduces to:

$$Cl = \frac{K_o A}{1 + K_o A/Q_d} \qquad (\#11)$$

For a substance of sufficiently large molecular weight to be characterized by a small $K_o A$, the above equation can be further simplified. If, for example, $K_o A$ equals 15, the quotient $K_o A/Q_d$ will be only 0.07 at dialysate flow rates of 200 ml/min, and this small number has a minimal effect on the denominator of the equation. Therefore, when $K_o A/Q_d$ is much less than 0.1, equation #11 can be further reduced:

$$Cl \approx K_o A \qquad (\#12)$$

For higher molecular weight substances, the membrane resistance constitutes by far the greatest fraction of the total mass transfer resistance [11]. Membrane permeability can then be substituted for the overall mass transfer coefficient in equation #12. It is important to realize that Equation #12 holds *only* if the restrictions described above are met. The ratios of $K_o A$ to blood and dialysate flow rates must be much less than 0.1. Hence, the approximation is valid only for high molecular weight species and is not a valid estimate of clearance for most commonly measured compounds.

Some discussion of solute clearance from the body is in order and has been discussed in the literature [12]. If the body is represented as a single solute pool, the removal rate of a substance may be described by the simple differential equation:

$$VdC_{bi}/dt = ClC_{bi}$$

This states that the rate at which solute is removed from a pool may be estimated from the volume of the pool and the rate at which the concentration is declining. It is equal to the blood-solute concentration times the rate of clearance. The equation may be integrated directly between the limits of time at the beginning and end of dialysis to yield:

$$\ln(C^f_{bi}/C^s_{bi}) = (Cl/V)t \text{ or } C^f_{bi} = C^s_{bi} \exp[-(Cl/V)t]$$

It is evident that the fraction of the original blood-solute concentration to which the final concentration will fall is a function of the dialyzer clearance, the volume of solute distribution, and the time on dialysis. Further, if these parameters are known, the final blood concentration can be calculated directly. The amount of solute removed during a dialysis may also be estimated:

$$M = V(C^s_{bi} - C^f_{bi}) = VC^s_{bi}\{1 - exp\,[-(Cl/V)t]\}$$

The amount of solute the patient manufactured will equal the solute generation rate multiplied by time. If the patient is in equilibrium during the dialysis cycle, the amount of solute so generated will equal the amount removed during dialysis.

$$\lambda t = VC^s_{bi}\{1 - exp[-(Cl/V)t]\}$$

This, in turn, may be rearranged to estimate the predialysis blood-solute concentration [12]. If the solute in question is of sufficiently high molecular weight to warrant the assumptions, equation #12 may be substituted for clearance in these expressions. The amount of solute removed then becomes a function of membrane permeability, the membrane area, and time on dialysis, and is relatively less dependent on dialysate and blood flow rate. For substances of lesser molecular weights, a more complicated expression such as equation #10 must be used for clearance.

Unfortunately, solute generation rates may not be constant; they depend on body size or surface area, dietary intake, and probably a variety of other ill-defined variables. A further theoretical objection to an analysis of this sort is the observation that the human body may not in fact be a single pool, even for small molecules. Data presented by Shackman and colleagues [13], for instance, suggest that a significant disequilibrium between intracellular and extracellular urea concentrations may exist in some patients after hemodialysis. This observation supports the thesis that the body consists of more than one pool with respect to urea. Nonetheless, this model is useful for purposes of illustration, and predialysis solute concentrations can be estimated if one is willing to accept the simplifications involved.

The concept of clearance and time on dialysis has been described in an empirical sense by Gotch [14] to evaluate the amount of dialysis to which a patient is exposed. Here, total weekly clearance for a solute in question is estimated from an empirical determination of dialyzer clearance (as determined by equation #8, for instance) and the fraction of time for which a patient is dialyzed during the week. This seems to be a reasonable description of the quantity of dialysis a patient is receiving and can be easily estimated for solutes of varying molecular size.

PRESSURES AND FLOWS

Internal pressures and blood flow rates are intimately related during the operation of a hemodialyzer as seen from Poiseuille's law [15]. The pressure drop across the blood compartment of a dialyzer is obtained by simple subtraction:

$$\Delta P_b = P_{bi} - P_{bo}$$

Poiseuille's law states that this pressure drop is a function of the length of the dialyzer, the viscosity of the perfusing solution, the number of passages, some function of the average cross-sectional area of the passages, and the blood flow rate:

$$\Delta P_b = \frac{\eta \, l}{n} Z \, Q_b \qquad (\#13)$$

Z represents the function of the average blood path cross-sectional area, and for circular passages:

$$Z = \frac{1}{\pi r^4} \times 10^{-4}$$

For rectangular passages, the widths of which are very small compared to the heights:

$$Z = \frac{1.5}{w^3 h} \times 10^{-4}$$

If the system is rigid and the fluid is Newtonian, the relationship between pressure drop and blood flow is obviously linear. It is directly proportional to the length of the passage and viscosity of the fluid and inversely proportional to the number of blood passages and a function of their cross-sectional area. The cross-sectional area is important insomuch as $\Delta P_b/Q_b$ will increase as a power function as this area decreases. Inordinately high pressure is required to yield a given blood flow rate with small areas, therefore, or flow is reduced to a very low level for a given pressure source.

Blood is an anomalous fluid and its viscosity is not constant. Viscosity tends to increase with increasing hematocrit levels [16] and change with the dimensions of the passages and operating rates of shear. However, a useful estimating value in patients with chronic renal failure who are usually anemic is 0.02 to 0.03 poise [17]. Further complicating the matter is the fact that a blood passage may be compliant and its dimensions not stable under all operating conditions. As the internal pressure of the dialyzer changes, the blood compartment may expand or contract and the cross-sectional area of the blood path may change. One can see from equation #13 that the pressure drop to blood flow ratio, often referred to as the blood flow resistance, changes as this cross-sectional area changes. Figure 3 illustrates the pressure drop versus blood flow curves obtained from a rigid capillary system, the internal dimensions of which do not change with changing internal pressures. A similar curve from a more compliant coil device is shown for comparison. The relationship of pressure drop to blood flow is linear in the rigid system. In the more compliant device, the increasing internal pressures that attend higher blood flow rates distend the blood compartment, resulting in a decreasing $\Delta P_b / Q_b$ with increasing blood flow rates.

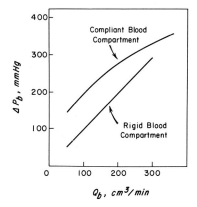

Fig. 3. Relationship between pressure drop and blood flow for a device with a rigid blood compartment and for a device with a compliant blood compartment.

DYNAMIC VOLUMES

A system's compliance may be defined as the change in internal volume per unit change in transmembrane pressure. The transmembrane pressure is the simple pressure difference across the membrane and is represented by the difference between the average pressures in the blood and dialysate compartments.

$$\Delta \bar{P}_m = \frac{\Delta P_b}{2} + P_{bo} - \bar{P}_d = \frac{P_{bi} + P_{bo}}{2} - \bar{P}_d \qquad (\#14)$$

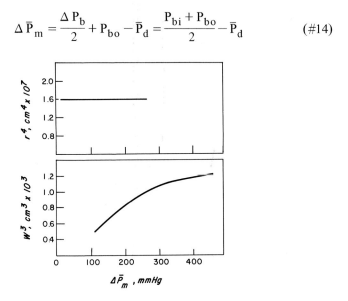

Fig. 4. Average cross-sectional dimension (raised to an appropriate power) for a rigid blood compartment on the top (hollow fiber kidney) and for a compliant blood compartment on the bottom (twin coil).

Figure 3 illustrates that $\Delta P_b/Q_b$ may decrease with increasing flow rates, likely due to the increasing transmembrane pressures that attend increasing blood flow rates. Figure 4 illustrates the stability of internal geometry in noncompliant devices and the relative instability in more compliant devices in response to changes in transmembrane pressure. Functions of radius or channel width may be estimated from $\Delta P_b/Q_b$ by rearranging equation #13. The figure to the right represents the capillary device, and the radius of the capillaries does not change significantly with increasing transmembrane pressure. However, the channel width of the more compliant dialyzer shown on the right increases significantly with increasing transmembrane pressure. As this width increases, the volume of the device expands $(V = whl)$. Unfortunately, the degree of volume expansion may be different in individual devices, even within a particular design or model. Figure 5 illustrates the compliance curves of three different similar-model twin-coils, and it is evident that the expansion of these may vary markedly from unit to unit.

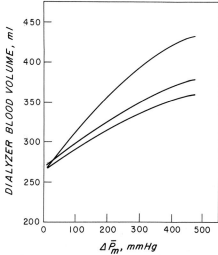

Fig. 5. Compliance curves illustrated by volume of hemodialyzers as a function of average transmembrane pressures. The three curves were obtained on different exchangers of similar model (twin coil) and indicate that marked differences in compliance may exist between individual devices of similar model.

At the start of any dialysis, when blood flow rate is increased the volume of a compliant dialyzer will expand in proportion to the increasing transmembrane pressure. This will effect a net shift of blood from patient to dialyzer, the quantity of which will be different for different dialyzers. The magnitude of this effect will obviously depend on the device's compliance and basic priming volume (dialyzer volume at very low transmembrane pressure).

FLUID REMOVAL

Fluid removal is an important aspect of clinical hemodialysis. Removal of excess fluid is essential for the control of heart failure and hypertension, but excessive fluid removal can lead to hypotension and an uncomfortable treatment. The rate of fluid removal is often referred to as the ultrafiltration rate. The two components of total fluid removal rate are that due to a hydrostatic transmembrane pressure gradient and that due to the osmotic transmembrane pressure gradient [18]:

$$Q_f = Q_{f,h} + Q_{f,osm}$$

The rate of fluid removal due to hydrostatic pressure is a function of the dialyzer's specifications, the ultrafiltration coefficient, and the surface area:

$$Q_{f,h} = L_h A \, \Delta \bar{P}_{m,h}$$

For any given device, however, the hydrostatic ultrafiltration rate is a simple linear function of transmembrane pressure [19]. This is illustrated in Figure 6 for an experimental hollow fiber artificial kidney.

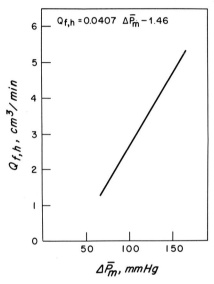

Fig. 6.   Hydraulic ultrafiltration rate plotted as a function of average transmembrane pressure. A straight line of relationship is observed.

Total fluid removal can be predicted most accurately by measuring average transmembrane pressure (equation #14) during clinical dialysis and multiplying by $L_h A$ and time. Many dialysis centers do not routinely measure both inlet and outlet pressures, however, and nomograms for predicting $Q_{f,h}$ from clinical data or equations for their construction have been published [20-23].

Fluid loss due to osmotic gradients is more difficult to estimate. The net *effective* transmembrane osmotic pressure determines $Q_{f,osm}$. The total gradient is the sum of the mean osmolar gradients expressed in millimeters of mercury for each molecular species multiplied by the appropriate reflection coefficient of the membrane for the molecule in question:

$$\Delta\overline{P}_{m,osm} = \frac{1}{n}\Sigma(\Delta\overline{C}_{osm}\sigma)_i = (\Delta\overline{C}_{osm}\sigma)_1 + (\Delta\overline{C}_{osm}\sigma)_2 + \cdots + (\Delta\overline{C}_{osm}\sigma)_n$$

Reflection coefficients are thermodynamically defined [18] and are estimated by comparing the solvent flux induced by a hydrostatic force across the membrane to that induced by a particular osmotic force (L_{osm}/L_h). For these purposes, then, it is an ''efficiency'' parameter. The coefficient is related to the permeability of the membrane to the solute in question. Coefficients of one are associated with complete impermeability and full osmotic effect while coefficients of zero are associated with complete permeability and no osmotic effect.

Under most circumstances, the *effective* osmotic pressures of blood and dialysate nearly balance, and the net effective transmembrane osmolar gradient approaches zero or is small compared to the hydrostatic gradient. However, if blood-solute concentration is extremely high (as is the case with glucose in a diabetic patient, or with mannitol after large quantities have been administered), the osmotic effect could slightly diminish fluid loss. Glucose, on the other hand, has been added to dialysate in high concentrations to enhance fluid loss during clinical hemodialysis. One may predict the magnitude of this effect from a knowledge of the ultrafiltration coefficient of the dialyzer, the reflection coefficient of the membrane for glucose, an estimate of the inlet blood-glucose concentration, the dialyzer area, and the overall mass transfer coefficient for glucose. From these parameters, equations have been derived which predict $Q_{f,osm}$ from dialysate-glucose concentration and blood flow rate [24]. Nomograms such as Figure 7 may then be constructed for any given dialyzer design.

BLOOD RECOVERY

Since anemia is a worrisome symptom of chronic renal failure, blood loss as a result of hemodialytic therapy should be minimized. Unfortunately, blood remains behind in the dialyzer at the end of a given treatment and may constitute a significant source of blood loss. There are two basic components to the quantity of blood that remains behind at the conclusion of a treatment. The first includes small clots within the device or red cells firmly adherent to membranes. This quantity of blood may be considered irretrievably lost—only the sever-

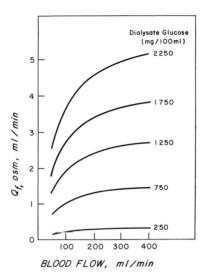

Fig. 7.   Nomogram for predicting the effects of increasing dialysate-glucose concentration on ultrafiltration rate for one twin coil design.

est washing can remove it from the dialyzer. The second component is that blood which could potentially be completely washed out of the dialyzer if sufficient volumes of rinsing fluid were used. Usually, a dialysis nurse or technician does not completely rinse blood from the dialyzer at the conclusion of a treatment because of the untoward quantities of saline this might require.

   If the hematocrit in the fluid being returned to the patient versus the reinfusion volume is plotted on semilog paper, a graph such as Figure 8 is obtained. The straight line portion of the curve can be extrapolated back to zero volume to obtain an "artificial" intercept H_a. For points beyond the inflection of the curve, the quantity of red cells remaining in the dialyzer may be obtained by:

$$RC = \frac{H_a v_{1/2} e^{-(0.693/v_{1/2})v}}{0.693}$$

Here, $v_{1/2}$ represents the half-volume of the straight line portion of the curve. The quantity of whole blood remaining in the dialyzer can then be obtained by dividing the red cell volume remaining in the device by the patient's hematocrit:

$$WB = \frac{RC}{H_p}$$

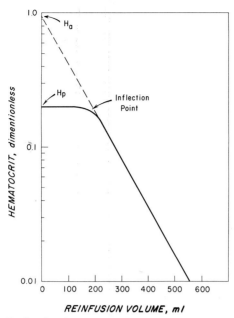

Fig. 8. Reduction in hematocrit of blood entering a patient during reinfusion is a function of reinfusion volume. The straight line portion of the curve shows an exponential decline and may be extrapolated to the ordinate.

This estimate applies only to potentially recoverable blood. It assumes that blood is washed from the dialyzer during reinfusion and that hematocrit in blood returning to the patient falls in an exponential fashion. Blood irreversibly lost within the device may be estimated from the difference between the pre- and post-treatment dialyzer volumes of noncompliant devices but is not included in this "washout" calculation. The total loss, then, is the sum of these two components.

CLINICAL HEMODIALYZERS

We do not intend to catalog or compare currently available dialyzers nor review the historical development of hemodialyzers. Rather, we mention several dialyzer types and characteristics to illustrate principles discussed in the preceeding paragraphs. An excellent catalog of dialyzer performance up to 1967 is available [4], and descriptions of various dialyzers' performance since then are available in volumes of the Transactions of the American Society for Artificial Internal Organs.

A hemodialysis system comprises two basic units. The first of these is the exchanger—that portion of the system in which mass transfer occurs. Its basic components are a blood compartment, a dialysate compartment, and an intervening semipermeable membrane. The second portion of the system is a device that delivers fresh dialysate of suitable composition to the exchanger. Exchangers in common clinical use today fall into three basic types—coil, parallel plate, and hollow fiber.

Coil Dialyzer

The performance of various coil dialyzers has been reviewed [20-23,25]. A coil is constructed from one or more membrane tubes which are concentrically wound with an intervening membrane support. Figure 9 illustrates the construction of such a device. Blood passes through the tubes, and dialysate is pumped at high velocity through the supporting structure over the outside of the blood conduits. The high velocity of dialysate flow and the turbulence created by the supporting structure are sufficient to reduce dialysate side, fluid-film mass transfer resistance to very low levels. Most coils are highly efficient devices that can yield a urea dialysance of up to 160 ml/min at a blood flow rate of 200 ml/min. They exhibit a high blood flow resistance ($\Delta P_b/Q_b$) at the hematocrit values commonly observed in our patients. Further, blood flow resistance may change as the coil expands or contracts with changing blood compartment pressures. Flow resistance will obviously vary according to the geometry of the coil in question (see equation #13). While under usual operating conditions an average value for flow resistance may be 1.0 to 1.5 mmHg/ml/min, values of up to 4 mmHg/ml/min may be observed with certain coils under certain conditions. If the coil outlet pressure is zero and the blood flow rate is 200 ml/min, the coil inlet pressure must be 200 mmHg if the operating flow resistance is 1.0 (see "Pressures and Flow" section). Coils operate then at relatively high pressures and a blood pump is required for their use.

The priming volume of coils may vary from 150 to 350 ml. They are compliant and as such may expand significantly during dialysis. Ultrafiltration rates tend to be relatively high because of the high blood compartment pressures attending clinical use. These two factors may lead to a hemodynamically unstable treatment. Nonetheless, coils are efficient and easy to use. They have been and continue to be a mainstay of hemodialysis therapy.

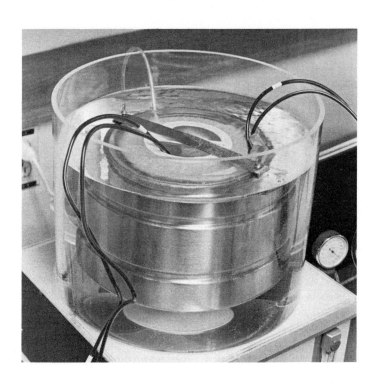

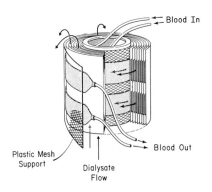

Blood In

Plastic Mesh
Support

Dialysate
Flow

Blood Out

Fig. 9. Photograph (top) and schematic diagram (bottom) of coil-type device.

Parallel Plate

Parallel plate exchangers were among the earliest dialyzers used clinically, and a variety of permutations on the basic design have been described. A dialyzing membrane is stretched over a supporting structure. Another membrane is placed on top of the first and blood ports are placed at both ends of the dialyzer between the membranes. Another support is placed on top of the second membrane. Blood flows between the membranes while dialysate flows between the supporting structures and a membrane. Supporting structures are of various designs and the number and configurations of tiers varies from device to device. The performance of earlier parallel plate dialyzers has been well reviewed [4]. The mass transfer performance of these devices has not been as impressive as that observed with coils. Generally, the number of hours of dialysis needed in a week to achieve the same clinical result has been greater using parallel plate dialyzers than using coil devices. One possible reason for the disappointing performance of these devices may be the channeling of dialysate with poor distribution over the membrane surface and a high dialysate side mass transfer resistance. Further, portions of membrane may abut the supporting structures resulting in loss in effective dialyzing surface area [26]. Certain designs have improved dialysate distribution and enhanced clearance of solute [27-29]. Nonetheless, dialysance of small molecules such as urea with these devices at blood flow rates of 200 ml/min is only 120 to 130 ml/min—less than that observed with coil-type exchangers.

Blood flow resistances in parallel plate dialyzers are usually small so that they can be operated without a blood pump when used in a patient with an arteriovenous shunt. $\Delta P_b/Q_b$ is usually in the range of 0.1 mmHg/ml/min—a factor of 10 less than coil-type dialyzers. Blood compartment pressures are low as compared to those of coil dialyzers. Transmembrane pressure may nonetheless be increased by applying a vacuum to the dialysate compartment. This maneuver usually permits adequate ultrafiltration rates. However, if the negative pressure applied to the dialysate compartment is reduced to very low levels, only minimal ultrafiltration may be achieved. The versatility is a decided advantage. Blood compartment priming volumes are usually low, ranging from 100 to 150 ml, and while the blood compartment is compliant, dynamic volumes are usually less than these observed with coil-type devices.

Hardware may be somewhat bulky and inconvenient, and the necessity for stacking membranes between dialyses may be a disadvantage. This is particularly true for large-center dialysis units. Some prepackaged parallel plate dialyzers are currently available [30]. Figure 10 depicts such a device. Urea clearances are similar to those of other

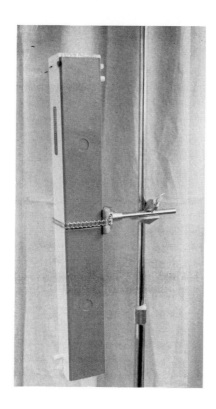

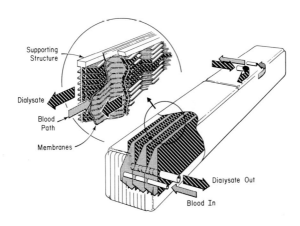

Fig. 10. Photograph (top) and schematic diagram (bottom) of self-contained parallel plate hemodialyzer.

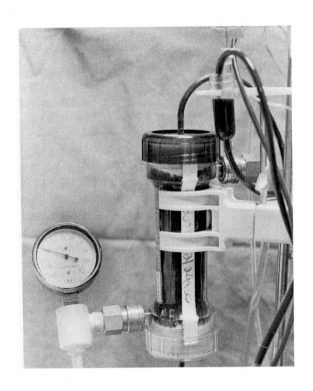

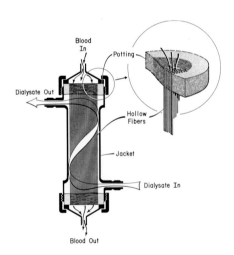

Fig. 11. Photograph (top) and schematic diagram (bottom) of a hollow fiber hemodialyzer.

parallel plate devices providing 1 square meter of dialyzing surface and are approximately 125 ml/min at a blood flow rate of 200 ml/min. Priming volume is approximately 90 ml, and dialyzer volume may increase up to 200 ml at higher transmembrane pressures. Blood flow resistance reported as 0.05 mmHg/ml/min is extremely low. Ultrafiltration rate can be well controlled between 0 and 12 ml/min [30]. Devices such as this seem to retain some of the relative advantages of other parallel plate dialyzers while solving many of the objections to their use.

Hollow Fiber Kidney

The performance of the hollow fiber kidney has been well described [31,32]. The device depicted in Figure 11 employs 10,000 to 15,000 hollow fibers with an internal diameter of 200μ to 250μ as a dialyzing surface. From an engineering point of view, this configuration represents an optimal dialyzer design. The narrow channels allow a minimum blood-fluid film resistance and a maximum surface area to blood volume ratio. The device has extremely stable dimensions and is, for all practical purposes, noncompliant. Internal blood volume is therefore stable and does not expand or contract with changing transmembrane pressures.

Mass transfer capabilities approach that achievable with coil-type devices. Ultrafiltration is predictable and can be controlled from approximately 0.5 to 12 ml/min. The most significant problem experienced with this device to date is clotting of the hollow fibers. While this is somewhat less of a problem than in the past [32], the problem still exists. Clotting leads to a reduced surface area and diminished mass transfer capabilities. Further, fiber clotting leads to loss of blood that cannot be returned to the patient at the end of dialysis. If, for example, the fiber bundle volume of a hollow fiber dialyzer is 100 ml and 10% of the fibers clot during a given dialysis, estimated irretrievable blood loss is 10 ml. In addition, some blood will remain in the device at the end of reinfusion, but this represents potentially retrievable blood. The total loss as a result of the procedure is the sum of these two sources, and recent observations [33] suggest that blood loss with hollow fiber kidneys may be inordinately high.

Dialysate Delivery Systems

Dialysate delivery systems may be classified into two broad types. The first of these is a batch system in which a concentrate or individual chemicals such as sodium chloride, sodium bicarbonate, calcium chloride, and magnesium chloride is added to water in sufficient quantity to bring the ionic composition of dialysate to the desired level. The prototype of this model is the tank dialyzer in which concentrate is diluted to a volume of 100 liters. Dialysate is pumped over the membrane of a coil exchanger and, after a variable period of time, the contents of the tank are drained and a new batch of dialysate is mixed. Figure 12 depicts such a system.

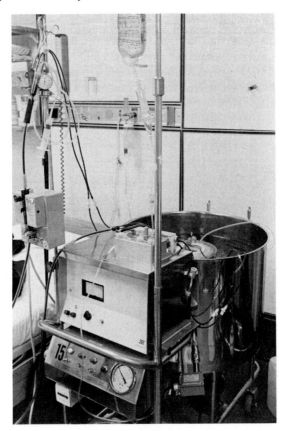

Fig. 12.   Typical tank-type hemodialysis system.

Another batch dialyzer is the so-called recirculating single pass system. Dialysate is mixed in a container and stored. It is pumped at a desired feed rate into a second reservoir containing the exchanger.

Within this second reservoir, dialysate is pumped over the coil in much the same fashion as in tank-type dialyzers. As fresh dialysate enters the reservoir, used dialysate overflows, enters a drain, and is discarded. The recirculating rate in such dialyzers may be 12 to 20 l/min, whereas the "feed-bleed rate" is variable and is usually 500 ml/min. Batches of dialysate may also be mixed and stored in tanks to be pumped or sucked over the dialyzing membranes of parallel plate or hollow fiber kidneys.

Dialysate-proportioning systems have recently found widespread clinical use. In these devices, dialysate concentrate is continuously mixed with water to be distributed over dialyzing membranes. Hemodialysis concentrate is mixed with fresh water—usually in a ratio of 1:35—by a pump. The pumps used by manufacturers of these devices vary. A water-driven reciprocating piston pump is commonly used, however other systems employ roller pumps that are controlled by the output of a conductivity cell. These proportioning systems, which are commonly used to supply a single exchanger, are also equipped with a variety of safety and hazard-detection devices such as conductivity cells and hemoglobin detectors downstream from the exchanger.

Large proportioning systems capable of preparing fresh dialysate for dialysis units of up to 20 beds are also available. Dialysate is then piped through the walls to individual bedside modules. In large units this arrangement saves nurse and technician time as well as space.

We will not embark upon a detailed discussion of various proportioning systems and the fail-safe devices with which they are equipped. Dialysate delivery hardware is changing at a sufficiently rapid rate to render any such discussion promptly out of date. Before purchasing such equipment, one must investigate carefully the pros and cons of each system under consideration. Probably the greatest factor in such a decision is the availability of technical service and support in the case of equipment malfunction. There can be no greater inconvenience or hazard than to have malfunctioning equipment with no technically competent representative of the manufacturer available to repair it.

Sorbents recently have received attention in the therapy of chronic renal failure. Much work has dealt with the oral ingestion of these materials or with sorbent hemoperfusion. Nevertheless, these procedures must be considered experimental and their therapeutic efficacy has yet to be demonstrated. Sorbents have also been used to regenerate dialysate, and a system employing this technique has been used clinically [34,35]. In essence, used dialysate is exposed to urease which converts urea into ammonia and carbon dioxide. The dialysate then passes over various sorbents including zirconium phosphate, zirconium oxide, and charcoal. Charcoal adsorbs many compounds that may be of importance in uremia, such as indican, phenols, uric acid, and creatinine. Unfortunately, charcoal does not adsorb urea well—hence the need for an active urease system to convert urea to ammonia and carbon dioxide. Ammonia is adsorbed by zirconium phosphate and is efficiently removed from dialysate. Zirconium oxide adsorbs phosphate. However, zirconium phosphate also takes up calcium and magnesium, and these ions must be added to the regenerated dialysate downstream from the sorbents. Hemodialysis has been performed in humans using as little as 1 liter of dialysate which is continuously regenerated [35]. The system shows promise and may provide a simple, portable dialysate delivery system.

REFERENCES

1. Wolf, L., Jr., Zultzman, S.: Optimum geometry for artificial kidney dialyzers. Ch E Prog Symp Series 84:104, 1968.
2. Wolf, A.V., Kemp, D.G., Kiley, J.E., et al.: Artificial kidney function, kinetics of hemodialysis. J Clin Invest 30:1062, 1951.
3. Michaels, A.S.: Operating parameters and performance criteria for hemodialyzers and other membrane-separation devices. Trans Am Soc Artif Intern Organs 12:387, 1966.
4. Colton, C.K.: A review of the development and performance of hemodialyzers. Cont. #PH-43-66-491; Artificial kidney–Chronic Uremia Program; Federal Clearing House Accession #PB 182, May, 1967.
5. Gotch, F.A., Autian, G., Colton, C., et al: Evaluation of Hemodialyzers, Report to Artificial Kidney–Chronic Uremia Program NIAMD, DHEW Publ. No. (NIH) 1972, pp 72-103.
6. Pappenheimer, J.R.: The passage of molecules through capillary walls. Physiol Rev 33:387, 1953.
7. Hamilton, R., Ford, C., Colton, C., et al: Blood cleansing by diafiltration in uremic dog and man. Trans Am Soc Artif Intern Organs 17:259, 1971.
8. Clark, W.M.: Topics in Physical Chemistry. Baltimore, Williams & Wilkins, 1952, pp 127-219.
9. Kays, W., London, A.: Compact Heat Exchangers. Palo Alto. The National Press, 1955, pp 7-24,33.
10. Renkin, E.M.: The relation between dialysance, membrane area, permeability and blood flow in the artificial kidney. Trans Am Soc Artif Intern Organs 2:102, 1956.
11. Colton, C.K.: Permeability and transport studies in batch and flow dialyzers with applications to hemodialysis, thesis. Mass Inst Tech, Cambridge, 1969.
12. Babb, A.A.L., Popovich, R.P., Christopher, T.G., et al: The Genesis of the square meter hour hypothesis. Trans Am Soc Artif Intern Organs 17:81, 1971.

13. Shackman, R., Chisholm, G., Holden, A., et al: Urea distribution in the body after hemodialysis. Br Med J 2:355, 1962.
14. Gotch, F.A.: Personal communications.
15. Bird, R.G., Stewart, W.E., Lightfoot, E.M.: Transport Phenomenon. New York, John Wiley and Sons, Inc, 1960, pp 42-54.
16. Pirofsky, B.: The determination of blood viscosity in man by a method based on Poiseuille's law. J Clin Invest 32:292, 1953.
17. Rand, P.W., LaCombe, E., Hunt, H.E., et al: Viscosity of normal human blood under normothermic and hypothermic conditions. J Appl Physiol 19:117, 1964.
18. Katchalsky, A., and Curran, P.F.: Nonequilibrium Thermodynamics in Biophysics. Cambridge, Harvard Univ Press, 1965, pp 117-126.
19. Nolph, K.D., Fox, M., Maher, J.: Factors affecting the ultrafiltration rate from standard dialysis coils. Trans Am Soc Artif Intern Organs 16:487, 1970.
20. Easterling, R.E., Haig, O.G., Green, J.A.: The plastic mesh support twin-coil hemodialyzer: Ultrafiltration, volume, erythrocyte recovery and safety. Trans Am Soc Artif Intern Organs 14:114, 1968.
21. Lowrie, E.G., Hampers, C.L., Merrill, J.P.:Twin-Coil: performance and predictability. Trans Am Soc Artif Intern Organs 15:60, 1969.
22. Sweeney, M.J.: Mass transfer during dialysis. Proc Third Annual Contractors Conf. Artif. Kidney-Chronic Uremia Program, NIAMD, 1970, p 36.
23. Easterling, R.E., Schulz, M., Knepley, W.: Comparison of the hollow fiber artificial kidney with the coil dialyzers. Proc Clin Dial and Trans Forum 1:25, 1971.
24. Lowrie, E.G., Goldstein, R., Hampers, C.L., et al: Ultrafiltration rate due to added glucose during hemodialysis (abstract), 18th Meeting, Am Soc Artif Intern Organs 36, 1972.
25. Bergman, L.A., Basha, H.M., Gora, A.H., et al: The EX-01 Cartridge—experience with 800 dialyses. Trans Am Soc Artif Intern Organs 15:65, 1969.
26. Mrava, G.L., Webber, D.C., Malchesky, P.S., et al: Computerized data analysis of hemodialyzers by a standard protocol shows true effective membrane area. Trans Am Soc Artif Intern Organs 16:155, 1970.
27. Steinmuller, S., Horn, E., Hamilton, R., et al: Clinical evaluation of the disk cone dialyzer. Trans Am Soc Artif Intern Organs 17:273, 1971.
28. Gotch, F.A., Edson, H.: Clinical evaluation of the western gear high performance multiple point support dialyzer. Fourth Annual Contractors' Conf., NIAMD, N.I.H., January, 1971, p 44.
29. Edson, H., Keen, M., Gotch, F.: Comparative solute transport and therapeutic effectiveness of multiple point support and standard kiil hemodialyzers. Trans Am Soc Artif Intern Organs 18:113, 1972.
30. Lindholm, T., Gullberg, C., Akerlund, A.: Laboratory and clinical experiences with a new disposable parallel flow plate dialyzer. Scand J Urol Nephrol 13 (suppl): 4, 1972.
31. Gotch, F., Lipps, B., Weaver, J., et al: Chronic hemodialysis with the hollow fiber artificial kidney. Trans Am Soc Artif Intern Organs 15:87, 1969.

32. Gotch, F., Sargent, J., Keen, M., et al: Development and long-term clinical evaluation of a thromboresistant hollow fiber kidney. Trans Am Soc Artif Intern Organs 18:135, 1972.
33. Kennedy, A.C.: Blood loss in regular dialysis. (abstract) Plenary Sessions and Symposia, Fifth Int. Cong. Nephrology, Oct. 1972, p 62.
34. Gordon, A., Greenbaum, M., Marantz, L., et al: A sorbent based low volume recirculating dialysate system. Trans Am Soc Artif Intern Organs 15:347, 1969.
35. Gordon, A., Better, O., Greenbaum, M., et al: Clinical maintenance hemodialysis with a sorbent-based, low volume dialysate regeneration system. Trans Am Soc Artif Intern Organs 17:253, 1971.

APPENDIX

SYMBOLS	DEFINITION	UNITS
A	Surface area	cm²
C	Concentration	mg/ml or mM/ml
Cl	Clearance	ml/min
D	Dialysance	ml/min
D'	Diffusion coefficient	cm²/min
H	Hematocrit (as a fraction)	dimensionless
K	Permeability, mass transfer coefficient	cm/min
L	Ultrafiltration coefficient	ml/min/mmHg/cm²
M	Mass	mg or mM
N	Solute flux	mg/min or mM/min
P	Pressure	mm Hg
Q	Flow rate or water flux	ml/min
R	Mass transfer resistance	min/cm
RC	Red Cells	ml
WB	Whole Blood	ml
V	Volume of distribution	ml
Z	A function of cross-sectional area	cm⁴
h	Long dimension of a rectangle	cm
l	Length	cm
n	Number of channels	—
r	Radius	cm
s	Sieving coefficient	dimensionless
t	Time	minutes
t'	Thickness	cm
v	Volume of reinfusion	ml
w	Short of dimension of a rectangle	cm
λ	Solute generation rate	mg/min
σ	Reflection coefficient	dimensionless
Δ	A gradient	—
η	Viscosity	poise

APPENDIX (continued)

SUBSCRIPTS

a   An intercept
b   Blood
d   Dialysate
f   Filtrate
h   Hydraulic
i   Inlet
m   Membrane
o   Outlet (with C) or Overall (with R or K)
p   Patient
osm   Osmolar

SUPERSCRIPTS

f   Final
s   Start

OTHER SYMBOLS

—   A bar over any other symbol indicates a mean but not
          necessarily an arithmetic mean.

2
Anatomy of an Artificial Kidney Unit

GENERAL PHYSICAL REQUIREMENTS

There have been considerable changes in the types of facilities required for hemodialysis in the last few years. When dialysis was initially proposed, all treatment was performed in the acute general hospital [1]. With the subsequent development of home dialysis [2, 3], part of the artificial kidney unit in the hospital was transformed into a "training unit" which by necessity had separate characteristics and requirements. Perhaps out of sequence, but equally as independent, has been the development of the "satellite" or out-of-hospital dialysis unit [4]. This unit may or may not be located in or adjacent to a hospital or medical facility. Since each of these types of dialysis units has different purposes, one must carefully evaluate the aims of the proposed artificial kidney program when planning and organizing the dialysis unit.

Many large dialysis-transplantation programs incorporate a combination of acute hospital, home dialysis training, and out-of-hospital (satellite) units. When these facilities are separate, each dialysis unit can be specifically designed. For instance, the hospital's unit—which in addition to caring for sick inpatients, serves as a backup for out-of-hospital and home dialysis programs—must be equipped to provide care for the acutely ill patient. This is especially true in instances in which an active transplantation program is a part of the overall care. We have found it essential in this situation to allow adequate room between dialyzing stations and to have each station equipped with oxygen, suction, and specific electrical outlets for the use of specialized bedside medical monitoring equipment. A unit constructed for efficient outpatient care would be unsuitable for the demands exerted on the acute hospital dialysis unit.

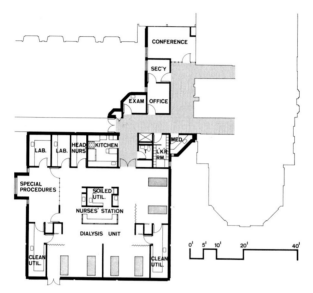

Fig. 1. Hospital dialysis unit that performs primarily "acute" dialyses. The space between dialysis beds is greater than is ordinarily required. The nursing station is not utilized for supervision of patient care, since most individuals dialyzed here require closer "one on one" supervision. In accordance with the requirements of an academic institution, a laboratory and a "special procedure" room are furnished.

Figure 1 shows a plan developed in 1967 for the Peter Bent Brigham Hospital In-Patient Dialysis Unit. While the nursing station is visibly accessible to all dialyzing units, the distance between the nursing station and the dialysis bed is too great to allow bedside supervision from the station. In other words, the nursing station is a central backup station, but the dialysis is done by a nurse or technician at the bedside. Since this unit is primarily used for acutely ill patients, large areas are open for free access of personnel and use of portable ancillary equipment. In our opinion, the in-hospital dialysis unit should offer a minimum of 140 sq ft per dialyzing station. Although the type of equipment used may influence this (i.e., hospital beds as opposed to lounge chairs), most of the space is required for nondialysis equipment and for access to the bedside.

An out-of-hospital dialysis unit may be constructed more compactly, since under ordinary circumstances it attends to more medically stable patients. For example, lounge chairs unsuitable for the "sick" inpatient may be ideal here. If home dialysis training is performed in an outpatient unit, a special area —100 to 115 sq ft per dialyzing unit under ordinary circumstances—should be assigned to this. Ideally this area should be away from the main line of traffic. Although home dialysis will be covered in a later section of this book, one cannot stress too strongly the need to train the patient in a systematic and organized manner. The amount of effort spent and the attention given to this early phase of dialysis will be amply rewarded in an uncomplicated and emotionally stable home dialyzing team.

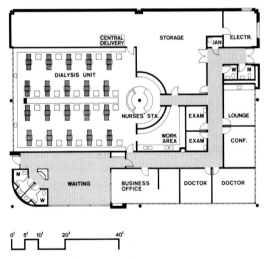

Fig. 2. An "out-of-hospital dialysis unit" also suitable for limited-care treatment. A waiting room is provided. Adequate storage space is essential and proximity of beds affords supervision by a minimum number of personnel.

Examples of out-of-hospital dialysis units in Figures 2 and 3 illustrate the prime concern—efficient use of patient space. Since the major fiscal expenditure in a dailysis unit is for supervising personnel, every planning effort should be made to maximize their efficiency.

The location of an out-of-hospital dialysis unit in relation to its back-up hospital varies, but we have found it most practical that they be nearby. This provides rapid transportation of the patient if an emergency occurs and allows the physician to be more available. Unless

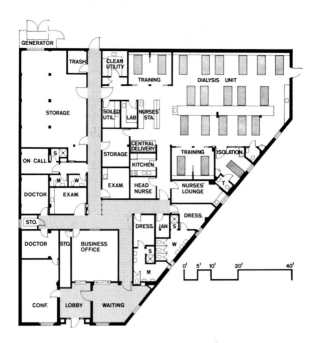

Fig. 3. An "out-of-hospital dialysis unit" that also has special areas for home dialysis training. These areas are located out of the mainstream of patient or personnel flow and can be isolated as required. In addition, a business office and an isolation room are also available.

the out-of-hospital facility is more convenient to the residential or office practice of the attending physician, there is some merit to locating it close to the hospital. In addition, the availability of public transportation for patient and staff should not be overlooked.

Other areas such as medication room, clean and dirty utility rooms, laboratory space, nurses lounge, conference room, and physician's examining room should be considered in planning the dialysis unit. When the unit is in the hospital, perfunctory administrative tasks can be handled centrally, but in out-of-hospital dialysis units these functions must be performed separately from the hospital. In addition, in the out-of-hospital unit, a comfortable waiting room should be provided.

In an out-of-hospital dialysis unit, if space is available, an "extra" bed or two should be available for patients who require attention after their routine dialysis. If the unit is operating at near capacity, such a holding unit is essential. After treatment some patients develop minor medical problems (e.g., hypotension, nausea, vomiting) that interfere with their immediate ambulation and subsequent transportation home.

PERSONNEL

Although many attempts have been made to establish definitive criteria for dialysis units, most of these efforts have been hampered by the diversity of available equipment and differences in philosophical attitudes concerning facilities. Certainly the *type* of program may have some bearing, for instance, on the number of nurses required, the ratio of registered nurses or licensed personnel to technicians, and the amount of physician time required. The acute hospital dialysis unit has requirements different from those of a low-keyed, out-of-hospital unit and from those of the out-of-hospital unit caring for recently discharged patients with acute medical problems. For this reason, we believe that the director of the dialysis unit is the key person assuring a successful and flexible operation. His credentials and experience are paramount. If he is adequately trained, most detailed decisions can be safely left to him. Unnecessary regimentation or regulations that may soon become obsolete (and are difficult to recind) can be avoided if the physician responsible for the dialysis unit is carefully chosen.

It is difficult to conceive that a dialysis unit providing comprehensive dialysis care (i.e., caring for both acutely ill inpatients *and* outpatients) could be directed by an individual with less than 1 year's experience (above and beyond that required for certification by the Specialty Board in internal medicine) in dialysis techniques. Ideally, 2 years of a nephrology fellowship should be required with at least 1 of those years spent directly with an active dialysis unit. Transplantation experience may be variably required, depending on the aims and purposes of the individual units. Satellite, noncomprehensive programs may be attended to by physicians with lesser credentials, provided they have easy access to "expert" opinion from a larger and more sophisticated program. The importance of the physician directing the dialysis unit cannot be overemphasized.

Moreover, no physician can be responsible 24 hours a day for the entire unit. Although only one "director" is required, backup physicians are essential. Under ideal circumstances at least two well-qualified nephrologists with dialysis experience should be jointly responsible for the operation of a dialysis unit. Physicians with less training but who have ready access to the director may be responsible for direct patient care. It seems to follow that any attempt to operate a dialysis unit of any size with only one physician will result in either total exhaustion of the physician or inadequate patient care. Obviously an active teaching program with research fellows and resident physicians in attendance can be a great asset to a dialysis unit and should be encouraged.

There is considerable difference of opinion as to whether or how long a physician should be in attendance during a dialysis procedure. Obviously, he is not present in the home dialysis situation. However, in in-hospital and out-of-hospital dialysis units, where patients may be maintained who have more complicated medical problems and who are incapable of being dialyzed at home, the medical situation may be different. In addition, in the home situation, a "one on one" consistent relationship between dialyzer and dialyzee results in predictable anticipation and experienced reaction to medical problems and patient idiosyncrasies. This type of familiarity between dialyzing pairs is impossible in a busy out-of-hospital unit where personnel vary (and thus specific physician participation is important in assuring consistency). We feel that although a physician need not be in attendance at all times during the dialysis in out-of-hospital units, he should be in attendance at the beginning of the procedure to see and examine each patient before or immediately after the initiation of dialysis. For some patients this may be excessive and unnecessary, but we believe that the majority of patients benefit from such attention. This has been borne out by our personal experience in an out-of-hospital dialysis unit operated in this manner that has shown a less than 6 percent per year mortality for 3 consecutive years, despite the fact that we utilize very liberal patient-selection criteria. This mortality is below the national average of approximately 10 percent [5], and in our opinion is directly related to the fastidiousness and frequency of physician attendance.

In the acute hospital situation, it may be necessary for a doctor to be present or readily available in the unit during the entire course of the dialysis. This is an individual decision and depends again on the nature of the patient being cared for in the hospital unit. We require that the physician be responsible for each dialysis to provide both medical care and emotional support—sometimes overlooked in a busy dialysis unit—to the patient and his family.

The nonphysician who is responsible for supervision, training, and overall management of personnel is also extremely important in a dialysis unit. A charge nurse who is mature, has the capacity for leadership, and is well versed on general nursing techniques and philosophy is essential. We have not found it necessary that she have a lengthy dialysis experience, provided she has some understanding of the procedure. If a dialysis unit is large and active, the head nurse's function is mainly administrative, and although she must involve herself in bedside management, she need not be the most proficient dialyzing nurse. This is in contradistinction to the requirements of the medical director.

As indicated previously, it is difficult to set firm rules as to the ideal number of registered nurses, licensed practical nurses, or dialysis technicians for a specific unit. This depends largely on the type of program provided and the type of equipment used. If dialysis bath changes are required, more personnel obviously are necessary. In units utilizing a central delivery system and no blood pump, a higher ratio of patients to personnel is in order. It is foolhardy to think that specific criteria can be universally applied.

We have found it practical to utilize nurse-technician "teams" to provide dialysis. This can be easily effected from a central nursing station. The nurse administers medications and other more sophisticated treatments. On the other hand, the technicians (several may be responsible to a single nurse) perform most of the details of the dialysis and may be more adept at such tasks as fistula-needle insertion (which requires a manual skill) than the nurse.

Every dialysis unit must have a satisfactory association with at least one surgeon—ideally but not essentially a surgeon experienced in vascular surgery. A general surgeon can easily master the surgical techniques required in providing an access to the circulation, and it is more important that the surgeon is available and interested than have definitive training in vascular surgery. In our experience most patients do better with and prefer an arteriovenous fistula. A number, however, still require an arteriovenous shunt. The problems attendant to these routes (discussed in another section of this text) may be acute and require the surgeon's immediate attention. While he need not be available 24 hours a day, there are enough calls that under ideal circumstances it is desirable to have two individuals who can "spell" each other.

Some dialysis units employ nonmedical "business manager" who supervises the overall operation. He may or may not be responsible for the fiscal aspects of the unit but certainly can be involved in such tasks as ordering supplies, establishing personnel policies, maintenance and housekeeping, and other functions usually left to administrators. We feel that such an individual can be useful, although he is not essential to the management of the dialysis unit. Many of these responsibilities usually handled by the hospital can burden medical personnel in an out-of-hospital situation when the dialysis unit is large.

As discussed earlier in this section, many of the procedures and policies applicable to a dialysis unit are individual and no sweeping generalities can be made. The type of equipment used depends on a number of factors, including the preference and prejudices of the director of the dialysis unit. Once a dialysis unit is in operation, however, it behooves the unit to have standard forms of medical practice, including manuals on all aspects of patient care. This is essential to providing uniformity of care in the unit, and it protects the patient from chaos and disorder if there is a loss of key personnel. Similar manuals should be available for administrative procedures relating to the unit.

REFERENCES

1. Scribner, B.H., Buri, R., Caner, J.E.Z., et al: The treatment of chronic uremia by means of intermittent dialysis: A preliminary report. Trans Am Soc Artif Intern Organs 6:114, 1960.
2. Merrill, J.P., Schupak, E., Cameron, E., et al: Hemodialysis in the home. JAMA 190:468, 1964.
3. Curtis, K., Cole, J.J., Fellows, B.L., et al: Hemodialysis in the home. Trans Am Soc Artif Intern Organs 11:7, 1965
4. Hampers, C.L., Schupak, E.: Long-Term Hemodialysis, ed 1. New York, Grune & Stratton, 1967, p 140.
5. Lewis, E.J., Foster, D.N., de la Puente, J., et al: Survival data for patients undergoing chronic intermittent hemodialysis. Ann Intern Med 70:311, 1969.

3

Access to the Circulation

Alfred P. Morgan, M.D.

Some chronic dialysis patients lead nearly normal lives. They feel healthy, enjoy working, and consider their commitment to dialytic therapy a tolerable necessity. Others are disabled physically and emotionally. Many variables contribute to the success or failure of dialysis treatment; they include such obvious factors as the original cause of renal failure, age, general life adjustment, and the presence of complications of the uremic syndrome or concurrent disease, but in addition, the apparently minor detail of making a connection to the patient's circulation is very important. The shunts and fistulas used for access to the circulation have a recognized symbolic importance to the patients, but their influence on the quality of life on dialysis goes beyond symbolism. Discomfort, disability, and metabolic consequences of marginal flow can tip the balance between satisfactory and unsatisfactory therapy.

There is no one ideal or best method for reliable and uncomplicated circulatory access. Instead, there is an array of possible choices. The list in Table 1 is not exhaustive but one of the included alternatives

Table 1

Primary and Secondary Methods for Circulating Access

Primary Methods

    Quinton-Scribner shunt in arm or leg

    Brescia-Cimino fistula in forearm

Secondary Methods

    External shunts

        Standard shunts in nonstandard sites: ulnar artery, peroneal artery, branches of the femoral artery

        Allen-Brown

        Thomas femoral

    Secondary AV fistulas

        Ulnar artery to basilic vein

        Brachial artery

        Lower extremity

        transpalmar

    Vein grafts

        Saphenous vein to forearm

        Saphenous vein in leg

        Xenograft and allograft veins

---

will fit the needs of any patient. Each method has advantages and disadvantages, and the choice of a method for an individual is made after considering the attributes of available methods. They are:

(1)   safety: the frequency and gravity of complications
(2)   magnitude: the extent of the surgical procedure required
(3)   delay: waiting time before use
(4)   duration: main time to failure requiring surgical revision
(5)   disability: functional impairment of the extremity
(6)   complexity: time, equipment, or skill needed for use
(7)   suitability: appropriateness of the method to the patient's individual vascular anatomy

The methods are primary or secondary. The primary methods are the Quinton-Scribner shunt [1] and the Brescia-Cimino fistula [2], and one or the other will be adequate for the majority of patients. These primary methods are simpler to establish and use, but there are a few patients for whom they will not work and a secondary method is necessary from the start.

Local conventions have some influence on the choice. Our unit leans toward the fistula, perhaps because passive flow dialysis is not used.

CHOICE OF METHOD

Criteria for initiating dialysis are discussed in another chapter. Once need for dialysis is definite, plans can be made for an access method. The patient is examined, the size and superficiality of forearm veins noted, and the patency of the ulnar and radial arteries verified by an Allen test. A radial pulse can generally be felt at the wrist after occlusion of the proximal radial artery. The pulse is transmitted through the palmar arches from the ulnar artery to the distal radial. Similarly, an ulnar pulse may be felt when that vessel is occluded. To prove true patency, the patient is asked to make a fist while the examiner occludes the radial and ulnar arteries at the wrist. Blood is expressed from the skin, and when the hand is opened, the palm will be blanched. If pressure on one of the arteries is released and if the vessel is open, cutaneous vessels rapidly refill and an almost immediate blush is observed in the palm. The maneuver is repeated with release of the other artery; either should refill the palm within a few seconds. Although an end-to-side fistula can be made to a vessel shown by this test to be the single major artery supplying the hand, it is a risk. Loss of arterial continuity when the fistula is made or following some later complication will usually cause ischemic symptoms. Use of a solitary artery for a shunt is even riskier because the vessel is always interrupted. It has been done when no reasonable alternative existed, and although tissue loss has not occurred, a cold or painful hand may result.

A radial artery to cephalic vein fistula is the preferred choice for primary access whenever adequate vessels exist. Complications occur less frequently with primary fistulas than with primary shunts. The procedure is minor, using local anesthesia in ambulatory patients, and takes about an hour. In the absence of complications the patient has full use of the extremity except during actual dialysis. Bathing, swimming, and all kinds of work are possible without special precautions. Most patients prefer a good fistula to a good shunt. Disadvantages of the fistula include necessity for venipuncture, some added cost for expendable supplies, and sometimes a necessity to wait for the venous limb of the fistula to dilate to useable size. Although more than half of the fistulas made can be used immediately and others need only a few days' wait for edema to subside, when usability depends on development of venous collaterals, waiting time may be weeks or even months.

If the best candidate for an arteriovenous fistula is a young male with muscular forearms and prominent veins, then the worst is an obese older female with small superficial veins hidden beneath a thick layer of subcutaneous fat. Patients with diabetes have trouble with shunts and fistulas. Diabetics usually have conspicuous atherosclerosis in both the radial and ulnar artery near the wrist, and their shunts tend to have poor flow and a high rate of failure. Diabetics may need a temporary shunt to begin dialysis but many are started with one of the secondary access methods.

The Scribner shunt in the arm or the ankle has the advantage of being immediately useable, and is the first choice in acute renal failure and when acutely decompensated chronic patients begin dialysis as an emergency. The disadvantages of shunts in long-term dialysis include a higher incidence of septic and mechanical complications; frequent necessity for anticoagulation; eventual failure by intimal pro- liferation or stricture; and most significantly, the disability associated with an external shunt. It requires daily care. Swimming and showering are only possible with waterproofing. Certain vocational activities are not possible. Although a shunt in the leg is somewhat more convenient, insertion of ankle shunts under local anesthesia can be uncomfortable and requires a week on crutches. Poor flow due to arteriosclerosis is more common in the leg than the arm.

When the primary methods for access are impossible or unap- pealing, the secondary alternatives are considered. If immediate hemodialysis is necessary, a nonstandard shunt may be the solution. The possible combinations are limited only by the surgeon's ingenuity, but most nonstandard shunt sites are too close to a joint or too hard to care for and do not last very long. For example, a shunt can be placed in superficial branches of the femoral artery and saphenous vein, or in the thyrocervical trunk. When the radial artery has been ligated, a short cannula can sometimes be accomodated in the distal stump of the artery. It is directed toward the hand and fills from the palmar arches. The ulnar artery is occasionally used even though the radial artery is not patent, as is the peroneal after ligation of the posterior tibial. Before either is used for the arterial limb of a shunt, it is of course advisable to observe the hand or foot for ischemia during a trial occlusion, but even when no obvious changes are seen, ischemic symptoms—usually swelling and pain—may occur later. Reconstruction of the artery after removal of the cannula was successful on the three occasions when it was undertaken, and probably should be done in this circumstance.

Two special shunts are available for use in sites where standard shunts do not fit. The Allen-Brown shunt (Fig. 1) is a length of 4-mm knitted graft glued to conventional shunt tubing. It permits an end-to-end anastomosis to be very close to the origin of the radial artery. The long-term patency rate has been inferior to shunts with internal cannulas, but this shunt has two attractive features: it allows use of what would otherwise be an expended vessel, and, like the Scribner shunts with straight tubing, it admits a small Fogarty catheter for declotting. This prosthesis may be used for the arterial limb of the shunt with a Scribner cannula for the venous side.

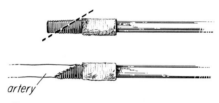

artery

Fig. 1.   Allen-Brown prosthesis. *Above:* Crimped graft is trimmed obliquely close to velour-covered tubing. *Below:* Conventional end-to-end anastomosis is made to vessel using 6- or 7-0 suture material. Magnification is essential.

The Thomas femoral shunt [3] is made to be applied directly to the femoral vessels (see Fig. 10, below). It offers immediate useability and high flow. The femoral vessels are usually available when no other sites remain. The important liability of the Thomas shunt is the threat of sepsis in the femoral triangle, a potentially life-threatening complication to be balanced against the immediacy of the need for hemodialysis.

Occasionally a nonstandard AV fistula will be useful. Any artery-vein pair can be utilized if a segment of superficial vein and a source of arterial blood are juxtaposed. Anastomosis of the basilic vein with the ulnar artery is the most frequent nonstandard combination, although the fistula that results from this anastomosis is less useful than one made with the radial artery and cephalic vein. The basilic vein is sometimes tortuous and usually thinwalled; the arm position during dialysis, elbow flexed and shoulder externally rotated, is awkward. Kinnaert found late thrombosis to be more common than for radial-cephalic fistulas [4].

Fistulas can also be made between the brachial artery and either

germicidal solution and draped. After local infiltration with 1% Xylocaine without epinephrine, a one-inch longitudinal incision is made over the radial artery beginning one inch proximal to the volar crease. A transverse incision is made over the cephalic vein (Fig. 3). Placement of the shunt closer to the hand would interfere with wrist flexion and with preservation of the dorsal branch of the radial artery. There is often an atherosclerotic plague in the more distal, more mobile part of the radial artery. The incision over the vein is chosen to avoid its bifurcation into volar and dorsal branches at the radial styloid (Fig. 3). The cephalic vein is usually visible or palpable, but if it is not it will almost always be found after the incision is made.

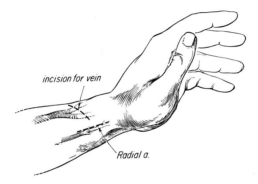

incision for vein

Radial a.

Fig. 3.   Incisions for Scribner shunt. Cannulation of artery is facilitated by longitudinal incision. The more mobile vein is exposed by small transverse incision.

The volar ramus of the radial nerve will be undisturbed if the incision is made directly over the radial artery. The subcutaneous tissue is divided and the vessel isolated. Its two accompanying veins are separated from it. The tiny posterior branches of the artery can often be cut a few millimeters from their origin and will retract without bleeding, but their avulsion from the parent vessel will cause a subadventitial hematoma. Subcutaneous pockets are made for the reverse loop tubing by blunt dissection (Fig. 4). It is important that the plane developed for the pockets be as deep as possible, immediately over the flexor tendons or muscle so that maximum thickness of tissue cushions the subcutaneous part of the shunt. The pockets should be generous. If they are too small, the shunt will extrude. The artery is ligated distally with 00 silk and a transverse arteriotomy made across exactly half its circumference. Polished, graded dilators are used to stretch the artery to 1.5 times its original caliber. With more dilitation

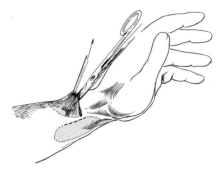

Fig. 4.   Pockets for reversed loop shunt are made generously
large and as deep as possible so that entire thickness of
subcutaneous tissue pads tubing.

the intima may split. The vein is similarly ligated and incised but can
be dilated to two or three time its original size. A cannula is selected
to make an easy snug fit with the dilated artery. Too large a tip will
push up a fold of intima during insertion. This is particularly apt to
occur with steroid-treated transplant patients and in shunt revisions.
If a short column of air is allowed to remain in the saline-filled tubing,
its pulsation can be observed during insertion. If the cannula should
be occluded by intima, the pulsation will stop and the tip can be withdrawn before insertion to its full length, and the intimal wrinkle can
be ironed out with a dilator or balloon catheter. A smaller tip can
then be inserted beyond the trouble spot through the same arteriotomy.
The tip is secured by a silk bridge, as shown in Figure 5. If the circum-

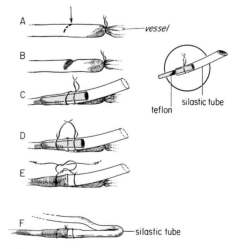

Fig. 5.   Assembled tip and tubing are secured by silk bridge.

ferential ligatures are tied down too tightly, they will dent the Teflon tip and cause early clotting. If a tip is bent during insertion or when the tubing is pulled through the stab wound, a permanent wrinkle is formed in its wall and it must be discarded. The stab wound made for exit of the tubing is placed to allow good axial alignment of tip and artery. The tubing must make a tight fit with the skin. A gaping stab wound that exposes subcutaneous fat will become crusted and then infected. A #15 blade makes a stab wound that is just the right size. The step formed in the shunt tubing should lie beneath the skin; if it is completely external, the shunt will extrude.

The venous limb is inserted in a similar way. A tip larger in relation to vessel size can be used, since the vein is more easily stretched and there is no danger of intimal dissection.

The tubing is cut to allow the connector to lie in the straight part of the external shunt. Flow is estimated by watching a small bubble travel through the tubing. If its motion is perceptibly pulsatile the shunt will probably clot and should be modified to improve flow.

The subcutaneous tissue is closed with absorbable sutures to create the thickest possible cover over the shunt. The skin edges are approximated with fine monofilament material.

Arteriovenous Fistula in the Arm

A primary fistula is feasible for at least three-quarters of new dialysis patients. The ideal patient is a male with prominent veins, his opposite an elderly diabetic woman with fleshy arms and tiny veins. With care and use of magnification, a patent anastomosis can be made between any artery-vein pair, but in order to be useful a fistula must be easy to enter with needles and provide 300 ml per minute of flow. More than half the fistulas made can be used immediately; others must mature before venipuncture is safe. In 61 fistulas made in 1969, mean time required before beginning dialysis was 5 days but the range was wide. The standard fistula is an end-to-side cephalic vein to radial artery anastomosis. It is preferred to the side-to-side configuration because it does not arterialize the veins of the hand, because mobilization of a distant vein is made easier, and because ligation of the fistula, should it be necessary, is simple.

A small transverse incision is used. The cephalic vein ordinarily branches just behind the radial styloid; the larger of the two branches is used and the other ligated. Veins are variable and other patterns may be found, but wheatever the local anatomy may be, some choice is made that will allow use of the largest vein available that will channel

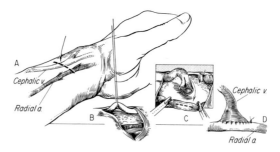

Fig. 6. Radial artery-cephalic vein end-to-side fistula.

flow directly into the cephalic trunk. The vein is mobilized and divided
distally. The proximal segment is dilated and spatulated as in Figure
6, and with bulldog clamps applied to the artery, a 0.4-cm linear
arteriotomy is made. Everting mattress sutures are placed in both cor-
ners and tied, drawing the vein down to the artery. Six- 0 or 7-0 suture
material is used. Running sutures complete the anastomosis. The length
of vein and position of the arteriotomy must be chosen so that the
venous limb of the fistula forms an easy curve without kinks or twists.
In closing the incision, some undermining may be necessary to prevent
compression or distortion of the fistula when the skin edges are brought
together.

Most fistulas exhibit an audible bruit and palpable thrill. Its intensity is related not only to measured flow but also to the accidental
hemodynamics of the anastomosis; nevertheless it is useful because
the patient can feel it and monitor fistula patency.

Saphenous Graft in the Arm

The side from which the saphenous vein is obtained is chosen
with regard to previous leg shunts, the presence of open wounds from
previous surgery, and the size of the vein judged by preoperative examination with the patient standing. A Scribner shunt in the ankle does
not prevent use of the vein above; in fact, the increased flow tends
to enlarge it. The vein is transplanted to the nondominant arm when
it is available for use. After skin preparation and draping, the leg is
positioned with the knee slightly flexed and the hip externally rotated.
A short transverse incision is made in the groin crease, centered on
the saphenofemoral junction. The vein is isolated. One or two of the
most proximal collaterals are preserved and others are ligated and
divided. The index finger is used to bluntly tunnel just deep to the
saphenous vein. Traction allows the vein to be palpated during this

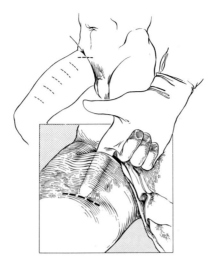

Fig. 7. Obtaining the greater saphenous vein: Ladder of short transverse incisions heals with better appearance and less contracture than longer longitudinal one.

maneuver. When the dissection has been carried as far as the finger can reach, a new transverse incision is made (Fig. 7). With exposure aided by a narrow retractor, branches within the tunnel are ligated and divided. If necessary, clips can be used and the clip on the venous side replaced by a tie later. The process is repeated until the vein has been freed to an inch or two below the joint line of the knee. The vein is divided proximally and distally and removed. Some attention should be given to noting which end is proximal and which distal: the saphenous becomes large at the knee, the presence of geniculate branches can simulate its appearance at the saphenofemoral junction, and the possibility of inadvertent reversed placement in the arm exists. After removal of the vein, it is cannulated and flushed with heparin saline. Then, aided by saline inflation, all branches are ligated flush with the main trunk and small leaks sutured. Pinhole leaks are stopped by 6- or 7-0 pursestring sutures placed in the adventitia. The occasional troublesome leaks that occur in the angle at the origin of branches are repaired without narrowing by forming a patch from the branch itself (Fig. 8). The final step in vein preparation is adventitial stripping. The adventitia is released, particularly around the valves, to obtain uniform caliber.

Attention is then turned to the arm. A transverse antecubital incision made through skin and subcutaneous tissue exposes the lacertus

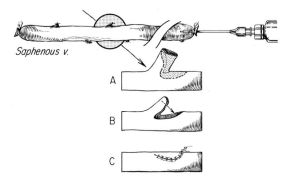

Fig. 8. Preparation of saphenous vein: Most troublesome leaks are in angle formed by branches and can be repaired without narrowing by patch formed from the branch.

fibrosus over the brachial artery medial to the biceps tendon (Fig. 9). This fascia is split to expose the artery. The medial antebrachial nerve may be seen: it can lie on the lacertus fibrosis or pierce it. The artery is separated from its accompanying brachial veins and a site for anastomosis selected somewhere above the origin of the radial and ulnar arteries. The venous anastomosis may be made either to a superficial vein or one of the deep veins. The deep system enlarges when many veins have been interrupted by previous shunts and may be a better choice than an antecubital vein that is larger but a veteran of many venipunctures.

A second incision is then made distally on the volar surface of the forearm; its position is determined by the length of vein available. A subcutaneous tunnel is formed, using a long pointed clamp, between the antecubital and the distal incisions. The tunnel is made very superficially. If the instrument forming it is allowed to follow the course of least resistance, the tunnel will be too deep. The vein is drawn

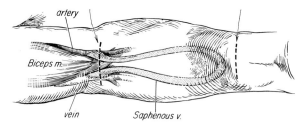

Fig. 9. Saphenous vein graft in arm: Here venous anastomosis is to cephalic vein. Distal counter incision does not lie over graft.

through without twists, its direction is reversed, and it is returned to the antecubital incision through a second tunnel forming a U-shaped loop. An end-to-side arteriovenous anastomosis is made, the venovenous anastomosis is completed, and the clamps are removed. The venous anastomosis may be end-to-end or end-to-side according to convenience.

It is possible to use a graft as a straight fistula between an artery at the wrist and a vein at the elbow, but only rarely is there an opportunity to do so. Patients who need a secondary fistula usually have had the distal arteries utilized for other access methods.

After wound closure, a posterior splint is applied to immobilize the elbow in 30 degrees of flexion. It is removed on the 3rd day. These grafts have been used for dialysis as early as 3 days postoperatively, but it is more usual to wait 7 to 10 days.

Saphenous Graft in the Thigh

When the saphenous vein is to remain in the thigh, the vein, still connected at the saphenofemoral junction, is removed from its bed and prepared as above. A counter incision is made on the anterior thigh and tunnels are formed for the loop. The femoral artery is exposed and its branches clamped. The end-to-side venoarterial anastomosis is usually made to the common femoral, but either the superficial femoral or iliac artery can be used. There has been no distal ischemia even in patients without popliteal or pedal pulses.

Thomas Femoral Shunt

The Thomas shunt antedates general use of saphenous vein grafts. Because sepsis in a Thomas shunt is hazardous, we have kept it in reserve as a last resort procedure, but there are still a few patients who have neither saphenous veins nor available sites for external shunts or internal fistulas; for them, a Thomas shunt may offer the best means of access to the circulation (Fig. 10).

A transverse incision is made in the groin. Thomas emphasizes that the approach to the femoral artery and vein be made by longitudinal dissection directly over the vessels to preserve a fibrofatty bridge containing the femoral nodes and lymphatics. This reduces the probability of postoperative lymph fistual and provides soft tissue separation of the two arms of the shunt. When the femoral artery, vein, and their branches have been exposed and tapes or elastic stays passed around them, a site is chosen. The relatively large vein offers no problem:

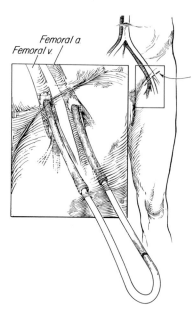

Femoral a.
Femoral v.

Fig. 10.   Thomas femoral shunt on the common femoral
artery and vein; other branches may be used.

the superficial femoral vein will easily accomodate the Dacron
prosthesis after some trimming of the fabric. However, even after
trimming, the adult shunt may be too large for a small superficial femoral
artery; the pediatric version should be available and will be used for
some adults. Even then it may be necessary to place it in the common
femoral artery.

With bulldog clamps on the artery, a l-cm arteriotomy is made.
The Dacron patch is trimmed to fit and sewn into the opening with
5-0 sutures. Caution is necessary when traction is exerted on the tubing
because the glued bond between tubing and cuff can be broken. When
the patch has been sewn into place, blood is allowed to run into the
shunt to clot the porous fabric. After a fibrin layer has formed, the
tubing can be filled with heparin saline and the venous half of the
fistula installed. It is instructive to attempt to pass a Fogarty catheter
through the shunt under direct vision. Its passage will at first be arrested
by the shelf formed at the junction of tubing and patch, but with the
use of a bent stylet and partial balloon inflation, the catheter can be
guided through the anastomosis. The tubes are then drawn through
separate tunnels to the anterior thigh. The position of the stab wounds
is carefully estimated. If they are made too close to the groin incision,

the velour-covered portion of the tubing will be extruded. A systemic antistaphlococcal antibiotic is given preoperatively and continued for 5 days afterwards.

CARE AND USE OF SHUNTS AND FISTULAS

Most shunts are used soon after their insertion; need for immediate hemodialysis is the most common indication for choosing this access method. Regional heparinization is employed for the first dialysis. If vasospasm causes low flow or high venous pressure, warming the arm and hand is helpful.

Care of the shunt between dialyses is a compromise. Measures that protect the shunt and prolong its life span often interfere with an arm function. Immobilization, for example, is good for the shunt but bad for the patient, and the usual compromise is to avoid repetitive motions like knitting and typing. Instructions given patients with Scribner shunts are:

(1)   Check daily for clotting;
(2)   Change daily dressing—wash shunt and skin with an antibacterial soap or an iodophor cleaning technique;
(3)   Keep the shunt dry;
(4)   Avoid carrying, lifting heavy objects, or vigorous activity with the shunt arm.

If clotting is detected, the patient usually comes to the dialysis unit, although home dialysis patients often declot their own shunts. Declotting begins with extraction of the thrombus in the external tubing, sometimes with the aid of a polyethylene catheter inserted into the lumen. The remaining thrombus can often be cleared by flushing with heparin saline. Too vigorous flushing can push the clot retrograde to the origin of the head vessels [7]. If flushing fails, slow intermittent injection of fibrinolysin solution may soften the clot and allow it to be aspirated. Once a shunt has clotted, unless there is a definite and corrected reason for clotting to have occurred and in the absence of contraindications to anticoagulation, the patient is begun on warfarin sodium.

Shunts frequently clot after a surgical procedure. Clotting can be prevented if patients admitted for surgery or some intercurrent illness have their shunts connected to a double syringe pump for the first few days. A flow rate of 1 to 2 ml per hour of heparin solution maintains shunt patency without measurable systemic heparin effect.

The arteriovenous fistula exchanges convenience between dialyses for a slightly more difficult process of connection to the machine. Two short thinwalled butterfly needles with attached tubing are used for the venipunctures. A single needle technique is also possible [8]. Quick and deft puncture of a large fistula may be done comfortably without local anesthesia. Most patients prefer that an anesthetic be used. Points of particular importance are alternation of sites of needle puncture are careful application of pressure after the needles are withdrawn to avoid occlusion. If a tourniquet is not used between the needles, a trial occlusion should be made of the segment of vein between them in order to be sure that blood is not being recirculated. The venous limb of an arteriovenous fistula does contain valves but they become incompetent as the vein dilates.

COMPLICATIONS

The overall complication rate for primary access methods in our patients is 12 percent. Most complications are minor, but a few are life-threatening. Almost all fall into one of three categories: mechanical, circulatory, or septic. Clotting is the most common complication; many of the others lead to it. The treatment of specific complications is a compromise between need for continued access and the consequences of the complication. Optimum treatment almost always implies loss of the access route, but sometimes a middle course is safe.

Mechanical Complications of Shunts

Erosion of skin overlying the subcutaneous part of the shunt tubing occurs most often in elderly patients with atrophic skin or when the shunt is placed in a sharply curved part of the arm. It often begins over the knot in the silk ligature securing the shunt. (The knot can be placed beneath the tubing when this complication is anticipated.) Erosion eventually exposes most of the reversed loop on a bed of granulation tissue. If kept debrided and clean, an eroded shunt can function for months but is mechanically insecure.

Shunt extrusion occurs when the subcutaneous pocket is too small to accomodate the reverse loop tubing. It may have been made too small or have become contracted by scarring. In either case, the subcutaneous loop is forced out through the stab wound. The cannula becomes angulated in relation to the vessel and the shunt will clot.

Sometimes tubing is accidentally rotated when the shunt is reconnected. It will usually be obstructed and clot but the twist can be detected by palpation and normal position restored. If declotting is successful, no permanent harm results.

Shunts may be avulsed accidentally. Less force is required during or after an infection. This accident has occurred when the shunt was being manipulated during a dressing change or dialysis, never spontaneously or during sleep. Patients need careful instruction in how to deal with a bleeding shunt and, even after instruction, may apply pressure over the stab wound where the bleeding appears rather than over the arteriotomy site where it originates. Stretched shunt tubing can also cause accidental bleeding. After many months of use the ends of the tubing that fit over the connector become inelastic and are easily separated. Old tubing should be trimmed occasionally.

The shunt that bleeds is a natural cause for concern. Some bleeding, measured in milliliters and occurring only during dialysis or when the prothrombin time is prolonged, probably originates from granulation tissue in the subcutaneous tunnel and is no real hazard. Bleeding vigorous enough to suggest an actual leak is usually associated with sepsis but does not always require revision of the shunt. Local pressure may stop it and, when stopped, the shunt can continue to be functional for weeks or months.

Mechanical Complications of Fistulas

Fistulas also clot, though not as frequently as shunts do. Usually the clotted fistula is thrombectomized or revised as described. However, when an arteriovenous fistula has been thrombosed by cardiac arrest or marked hypotension and the blood pessure subsequently restored, the fistula may be reopened by massage to dislodge the clot. There is an obvious hazard of embolism to the hand or the lungs. Whether to attempt this kind of closed embolectomy is a matter of individual judgment. The maneuver has been successful on several occasions when problems causing the low-flow episode made formal revision in the operating room impractical, and no harm resulted.

Local stricture is the most common mechanical problem of fistulas. Stricture is usually the result of repeated venipuncture in a single site. Short strictures can be treated by venoplasty. Uniform narrowing of fistulas, with thickening of the wall and mural thrombus formation (as evidenced by aspiration of thrombus from the lumen when the needle is inserted), is harder to repair. Anticoagulation does not seem to prevent it and usually a new fistula is necessary. Some fistulas develop the opposite problem, becoming excessively and uniformly large. The ectatic or varicose fistula does not necessarily show increased flow by plethesmography; it is simply unsightly. One large fistula did bleed spontaneously, but an ulcer was present over it and the bleeding was expected and prepared for.

Circulatory Problems of Shunts

Serious ischemia has occurred with shunts only in patients having a specific vasculitis. Minor symptoms are commoner. Patients who have had many arm shunts may have a detectably cool hand. Mild symptoms or even a degree of claudication can occur. The margin of safety is large but there is a limit to the devascularization of the hand that is tolerated.

Circulatory Complications of Fistulas

The question of high output failure due to arteriovenous fistulas is frequently raised. It has not been identified in our patients and probably does not occur with significant frequency, although it has been described [9]. It is a difficult variable to isolate. Congestive heart failure is certainly frequent in dialysis patients but is influenced by hematocrit, water and salt intake, and the quality of dialysis. The resting flow through a fistula is not a large fraction of normal cardiac output. Flow in a large, newly made radial artery to cephalic vein fistula is about 200 ml/min. In a saphenous vein graft it can exceed 300 ml/min. Branham's sign can be elicited only occasionally in patients with saphenous grafts.

Flow through the fistula can increase with time (it can also decrease, unfortunately) and measurements made of established fistulas show cardiac output changes in the neighborhood of 500 ml/min [10]. Concern with this aspect of fistulas is understandable. The hemodynamic effects of arteriovenous fistulas have interested physicians since John Hunter, and the circulatory consequences of larger traumatic or congenital fistulas can be dramatic; however, this feature of the smaller fistulas used in chronic hemodialysis is not significant by comparison to some of their other drawbacks.

The vascular steal is another theoretically reasonable circulatory complication of end-to-side or side-to-side fistulas. In one sense a steal occurs in every fistula with reversed flow in the distal part of the artery, and this is the majority. But, to be significant, this condition must not only be present but must cause symptoms, and this is unusual. Ischemic symptoms of the flow type apparently depend on the size and configuration of the anastomosis as well as on the patient's particular circulation. In one series [11], 7 of 8 patients experienced ischemic symptoms. Their mean resting forearm flow, measured plethysmographically, was over five times that of the control arms. This finding is probably explained by the size of the fistulas studied: 0.5 cm to 1 cm. Smaller (0.4 cm) end-to-side fistulas seldom increase limb blood flow more than three times and ischemic complications are rare. Larger more proximal fistulas made to the brachial artery caused ischemic neuropathic symptoms in 2 of 8 patients [12]. Brachial artery fistulas are a secondary procedure, performed after variable loss of the distal arterial circulation, and variable hemodynamic effects might be expected.

Still another circulatory consequence of fistulas in the upper extremity is an ulnar compression neuropathy or ulnar tunnel syndrome that follows dilitation of the ulnar artery [13]. Enlargement of arteries feeding a fistula is predictable; for a radial artery-cephalic vein fistula filled via the palmar arches, proximal dilitation may occur in the ulnar artery as well as the radial. The enlarged ulnar artery can compress the ulnar nerve as it crosses the carpal bones, causing ulnar hypoesthesia and intrinsic and hypothenar atrophy. This complication, like the occasional vascular steal, can be reversed by ligation of the radial artery distal to the anastomosis, converting the fistula functionally to the end-to-end configuration.

In a practical way the problem comes down to the analysis of hand symptoms when they occur and a decision to ligate or modify the fistula that is causing them. The severity, their reversibility, and the availability of alternative routes for access enter into the judgment. No firm rules are possible.

Septic Complications of Shunts

The shunt, always suspect when unexplained fever occurs in dialysis patients, is rarely proven to be the source of sepsis in the absence of local evidence of infection. Shunt infection occurs often enough, but it should be possible to demonstrate tenderness, redness, or drainage. Local infection can be treated with heat, an antibiotic, and sometimes drainage, and will subside. Oxacillin and vancomycin are currently used most frequently. The organism cultured has been usually but not always coagulase positive staphylococcus. Pseudomonas is occasionally cultured; one salmonella infection has occurred. Embolic sepsis, and of course cannula failure, are indications for removal of the shunt [14]. Successful treatment of local shunt infection reduces the shunt's longevity and may interfere with mechanical stability; tip avulsion occurs more easily in infected shunts.

Septic Complications of Fistulas

Local and systemic sepsis occur in arteriovenous fistulas although less commonly than in shunts. The clinical picture may be of septicemia without local signs of fistula infection [15]; the competing diagnosis is subacute bacterial endocarditis. More frequently a minor infection occurs first in a needle puncture site. It resolves, sometimes without treatment, but after a week or so the patient becomes febrile and the fistula tender. An aneurysm then appears and may enlarge rapidly (Fig. 11). Treatment by trapping and reanastomosis without excision is effective.

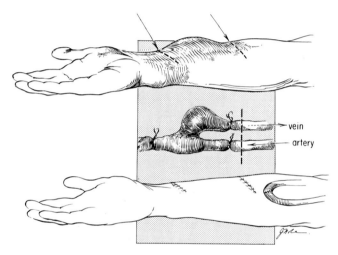

Fig. 11. Myocotic, anastomotic aneurysm in end-to-side fistula; these are treated by trapping and proximal reanastomosis.

METHODS OF REVISION

Shunt Revisions

Scribner shunts with reduced flow, clotted shunts, some infected shunts, and those which cannot be declotted will eventually need to be revised. The vascular cannula is removed and replaced in a new position about a centimeter proximal to its previous site. Usually only one side of the shunt is revised; the venous limb fails about twice as often as the arterial.

After shaving, germicidal preparation of the skin and shunt tubing, and infiltration with local anesthetic, the longitudinal incision over the artery is extended. Half of the old incision is reopened, and the new incision is carried about a centimeter into intact skin. If the venous cannula is to be replaced, a new transverse incision is made. The vessel is isolated, the old ligature cut, and the cannula and tubing withdrawn. To conserve vessel length the new arteriotony is made in the segment of vessel that was occupied by the old cannula. It is cleared of thrombus by flushing or with a small baloon catheter. Before a new cannula tip is pushed through the stricture formed by the tip of the old one, the vessel is dilated with graded vascular dilators. Vessels that have accommodated a shunt are visibly abnormal. Their walls are thickened and edematous and the intima of the artery is easily separated. Consequently, the tip size used is smaller than that chosen for a normal artery of the same caliber. Pulsation in the tubing is observed during insertion to be sure that intimal separation does not occur. A new pocket is formed for the reverse loop and a new stab wound made. In this way six to eight revisions are possible between wrist and elbow.

Revision of locally infected but well drained shunts can be successful. It is necessary to leave a little more room between the old and new sites. The old shunt is removed before final skin preparation and draping and the old stab wound draped out of the field. A systemic antibiotic is given until the new incision has healed.

After several revisions, the shunt may be so close to the elbow that flexion deforms the external loop of tubing, and a straight shunt is used. The tubing is led out through a tunnel directed toward the hand. Tacking sutures are placed between the ligature and adjacent tissue to prevent rotation in the tunnel. Shunts fitted with lateral flanges or wings [16] help to prevent both rotation and accidental withdrawal, but revision and removal are less simple. Eventually the shunt is so high that no further arterial revision is possible because the cannula would be occluded by elbow flexion. It is still possible to install an Allen-Brown shunt.

Phlebitis can make revision by simple advancement impossible. Phlebitic veins can be cleared of their contained thrombus but shunts made with them will ordinarily clot. In hospitalized patients or when the procedure is otherwise justified, a period of heparin infusion into the venous limb of the shunt allows the phlebitis to resolve and may salvage the vein. If a new vein must be found in the arm, the basilic or any other superficial vein may be used; in the ankle the lesser saphenous is a satisfactory alternative to the greater. Occasionally it will be advantageous to cannulate one of the deep veins that accompany the artery. They are small but distensible and useful. Revisions of the venous limb of a shunt need not always be made progressively closer to the elbow. Patent segments may remain between previous cannula sites, and when collaterals are adequate, retrograde cannulation of a proximal vein can be successful [7].

Shunt removal

Removal by open operation is more uncomfortable to the patient than removal by traction. The shunt is clamped and allowed to clot. Traction on the tubing will expose the ligature securing the shunt. It is cut and the entire shunt assembly withdrawn.

Fistula Revision

Fistulas may clot after a hypotensive episode or occasionally spontaneously during the hypercoagulable postoperative period, but clotting usually occurs after a traumatic venipuncture. The venous limb thromboses up to the arteriovenous anastomosis; in end-to-side fistulas the artery remains patent. If the fistula was satisfactory and if thrombosed for an identifiable reason, it can usually be cleared with a Fogarty catheter. A transverse incision is made 2 or 3 cm proximal to the original incision and the vein identified. The venous limb of the fistula becomes quite adherent to tissue around it and is easily damaged during dissection. If an attempt is made to free enough length to pass tapes around it or to apply bulldog clamps, the possibility of damage is increased. It is only necessary to expose a short length; flow is controlled by finger pressure applied by an assistant. It is usually not helpful to expose the anastomosis. A small transverse incision is made and the balloon catheter passed proximally and distally. It can be directed through the anastomosis and guided into either the proximal or distal artery (Table 2).

Table 2
Procedures for Revision and Repair

Shunts:	revision
Fistulas:	thrombectomy
	venoplasty of strictures
	collateral ligation
	proximal reanastomosis
	vein graft interposition
	exclusion of aneurysms

Variations of the procedure for fistula revision include placement of the incision over damaged or strictured portions of the vein with subsequent repair by vein patch or end-to-end interposition of a free graft. There is opportunity for variation and improvisation in the rejuvenation of fistulas impaired by local obstruction. For example, some can be improved by selective ligation of branches in order to direct flow into the main trunk. Proximal reanastomosis may be necessary if the original anastomosis has strictured. It may be convenient to make the new connection an end-to-end anastomosis, preserving maximum length of useable vein.

Other indications for fistula revision are mycotic aneurysms, which are treated by trapping, as in Figure 11, and the ulnar tunnel syndrome, which occasionally results from ulnar artery dilitation. The latter is corrected by ligating the radial artery between the end-to-side fistula and the hand.

Revisions and Secondary Access Procedures

Saphenous vein grafts occasionally require open extraction of thrombus or revision of the anastomosis from graft to vein or artery. Neither present any special problem. The Thomas femoral shunt may require revision due to accumulated pseudointima on the luminal surface of the patch and sooner or later will need to be removed. Because the velour-covered tubing stimulates a dense fibrous reaction, the complete exposure of the femoral artery, vein, and their branches is tedious but worthwhile. The shortcut of leaving the Dacron patch in place has been resisted since two episodes of femoral triangle sepsis, presenting weeks after shunt removal with retention of the prosthetic patch. No difficulties have been encountered in patients where the prosthesis was removed completely and a vein patch used for reconstruction.

REFERENCES

1. Quinton, W., Dillard, D., Scribner, B.H.: Cannulation of blood vessels for prolonged hemodialysis. Trans Am Soc Artif Intern Organs 6:104, 1960.
2. Cimino, J.E., Brescia, M.J.: Simple venipuncture for hemodialysis. N Engl J Med 267:608, 1962.
3. Thomas, G.I.: A large vessel applique A.V. shunt for hemodialysis. Trans Am Soc Artif Intern Organs 15:288, 1969.
4. Kinnaert, P., Vereerstraeten, P., Geens, M., et al: Ulnar arteriovenous fistula for maintenance hemodialysis. B J Surg 58:45, 1971.

5. Morgan, A.P., Bailey, G.L.: The transpalmar fistula for hemodialysis. Arch. Surg 104:353, 1972.

6. May, J., Tiller, D., Johnson, J.,: Saphenous vein arteriovenous fistula in regular dialysis treatment. N Engl J Med 280:770, 1969.

7. Gaan, D., Mallick, M.P., Brewis, R.A.L.: Cerebral damage from declotting Scribner shunts. Lancet 1:77, 1969.

8. Kopp, K.F., Gutch, C.F., Kolff, W.J.: Single needle dialysis. Trans Am Soc Artif Intern Organs 18:75, 1972.

9. McMillan, R., Evans, D.B.: Experience with three Brescia-Cimino shunts. Brit Med J 3:781, 1968.

10. Johnson, G., Jr., Blythe, W.B.: Hemodynamic effects of arteriovenous shunts used for dialysis. Ann Surg 171:715, 1970.

11. Bussell, J.A., Abbott, J.A., Lim, R.C.: A radial steal syndrome with arteriovenous fistula for hemodialysis. Ann Intern Med 75:387, 1971.

12. Matolo, N., Stevens, L.E., Chrysanthakopoulos, S.: Neurovascular complications of arteriovenous fistula. Am J Surg 121:716, 1971.

13. Morgan, A.P., Goldwyn, R.: The arm and hand in chronic hemodialysis. J Bone Surg Joint(Amer) (in press).

14. Goodwin, N.J., Castronuovo, J.H., Freidman, E.A.: Recurrent septic pulmonary embolization complicating maintenance hemodialysis. Ann Intern Med 71:29, 1969.

15. Levi, J., Robson, M., Rosenfeld, J.B.: Septicemia and pulmonary embolism complicating use of arteriovenous fistula in maintenance hemodialysis.
Lancet 2:288, 1970.

16. Ramirez, O., Swartz, C., Onesti, G.: The winged in line shunt. Trans Am Soc Artif Intern Organs 8:236, 1962.

17. Rao, V.P., Thomas, C.Y., Jr.: Retrograde cannulation of the cephalic vein for hemodialysis. J AMA 211:823, 1970.

4

Selection and Care
of the Patient

SELECTION OF PATIENTS

The methods currently employed in selecting patients for maintenance hemodialysis still vary from one center to another, and are still influenced by such factors as the personal philosophies of the physicians involved and the purpose of a specific dialysis program.

Whereas it was commonplace some years ago to employ selection committees on a routine basis [1], this is considerably less common now. The participation of lay members of a community in the decision-making process has ceased, and in those instances in which committees still exist they are composed generally of physicians trained in nephrology and most often directly involved in the management of patients with chronic renal failure. Regardless of the mechanism employed in selecting patients, the selection process ought to be directed toward choosing the most appropriate modality of therapy for an individual rather than determining whether or not to treat him. We have made it a point to develop a treatment program that will meet the individual needs of each patient.

Many factors enter into the selection process. Including the patient's age and intelligence, the availability of a suitable living kidney donor, the patient's motivation and ability to cooperate, the stability and support available to a patient at home, the presence or absence of a spouse and the spouse's occupation, financial resources, and finally but equally important, the patient's own preference. It has been our feeling, as well as that of most others, that the availability of a suitable and willing living donor would make transplantation the modality of choice for the young and middle-aged. Recognizing the hazards of arbitrary age limitations, we nevertheless tend to discourage transplantation in patients over the age of 55. Some patients, however, feel that the use of living donors is inappropriate and that transplantation should take place only when cadaveric material is available [2]. In our hands, when a suitable living donor is not available and the patient is seemingly an appropriate candidate for home dialysis, this then becomes the next preferred modality of treatment.

As experience with hemodialysis increases, the criteria determining patient acceptability continue to be liberalized [3-6]. Age, which once was thought to be an important determinant, is considerably less important now. We, as well as others, have dialyzed patients in their seventies and eighties with considerable success, and now several reports attest to the success of maintenance dialysis in the old as well as in the young [3,4]. The degree of success achieved with maintenance dialysis in the elderly population is notable and requires further comment. Over the past several years we have dialyzed 62 patients above the age of 60, and 11 patients over the age of 70. Despite their advanced years and the frequent presence of degenerative disease, these patients have done extremely well. Mortality in this group has been approximately 10 percent per year, which compares favorably with mortality for dialysis patients in general (i.e., 5 to 10 percent). In fact, in our experience patients above the age of 50 have done better as a group than patients below the age of 50. Although greater care and caution must be exercised in dialyzing patients in this older age group, the majority tolerate their dialyses well, follow directions and participate in their care better than younger patients, and are at least as motivated to survive.

Hypertension—particularly malignant hypertension—with significant cardiovascular complications was considered by some sufficient reason for patient rejection in the past [1]. This is no longer the case and with the judicious use of bilateral nephrectomy, drugs, and adequate dialysis, hypertensive cardiovascular disease is not a particularly difficult problem to handle and should no longer be regarded as a contraindication to maintenance dialysis therapy.

The association of diabetes mellitus with chronic renal failure has frequently precluded patients from receiving dialysis. This has been particularly true in patients who have had significant end organ deterioration as a result of diabetes. Here too, there has been considerable liberalization in the policy of accepting patients [5]. While some centers still reject patients with diabetes regardless of the severity of disease, age, motivation, or complications, more and more diabetics have found their way into treatment programs. Our policy has been not to arbitrarily exclude diabetics from treatment. The results, while not as good as those seen in the overall patient group, do seem to justify our decision. Of the 45 diabetics treated during the past 5 years, total mortality has been 30 percent and we have achieved success with several in home dialysis. In such instances, of course, the support and participation of the family is vital.

Lest we paint an overly optimistic picture of the long-term results achieved with diabetics, it is only fair to point out that some diabetics deteriorate quite dramatically and in several instances diabetic patients referred for dialysis never achieved stabilization and remained in the hospital until they died.

The diabetics problems above and beyond the control of diabetes may be numerous. The prevalence of infections at the site of venipuncture have made access to the circulation difficult at times. The inexorable progression of vascular disease has resulted on more than one occasion in amputation of one or both of the lower extremities. Autonomic dysfunction results in postprandial regurgitation and vomiting in some and may make proper nutrition extremely difficult. Several of our diabetics have had coronary artery disease accompanied by either arrhythmias or severe precordial pain during dialysis. We had to discontinue dialysis in one patient because of this. In another we discontinued dialysis at the family's request because of progressive deterioration and excessive patient suffering.

We have accepted for maintenance dialysis, patients with systemic lupus erythematosus, scleroderma, multiple myeloma, familial Mediterranean fever, and other systemic and disabling diseases. It would be foolish to establish standards for patient acceptability based upon disease category. Rather, we emphasize that each patient should be considered on an individual basis and not through the formulation of broad generalities. We believe that the burden of proof in the assessment of medical eligibility lies with the physician rather than with the patient and that the prime consideration should be whether or not the patient is likely to derive any significant benefit from the therapy.

Nonmedical factors influencing patient selection and perhaps patient well-being, as well as the modality of therapy to be used, are considerably more difficult to assess than is the medical evaluation itself. This may in part be attributed to the alteration in the psyche and personality stemming from uremia. It has been commonly observed that difficult and unmanageable patients may become pleasant and cooperative as their uremic symptomatology remits. It therefore becomes necessary to treat some patients and stabilize them emotionally as well as physically before any evaluation can take place. Similarly, it may prove difficult for the staff to get a clear representation of the family constellation during the initial introductory period. Problems do not always surface immediately and it is human nature for people to portray a picture of harmony and contentment when something less exists beneath the surface. Marriages which may initially appear to be ideal sometimes turn out to be quite fragile. Premature decisions based upon inadequate or hasty patient evaluation serve no useful purpose, and staff and patient alike are better off if adequate time is allowed for proper thought and reflection.

Once a patient has been found medically acceptable, the most important factor in his evaluation and subsequent course is his willingness and ability to participate in his own care. He should possess a thorough understanding of all aspects of dialysis and the management required for the patient undergoing maintenance dialysis. He should be totally familiar with the dietary constraints imposed by dialysis. Those who cannot, or will not, participate will almost invariably not do well. Although social and economic hardships may make cooperation and participation difficult, when patients are motivated to succeed they generally can, albeit sometimes requiring and obtaining assistance from the staff as needed. Motivation is a critically important factor in the broad determination of patient well-being. Patients who manifest vigorous interest in rehabilitation and demonstrate determination to return to their previous roles in society frequently are able to do so, while those who are unable to come to grips with the reality of their disease more often than not remain incapacitated. After receiving careful and repeated explanation of the irreversibility of their disease, some patients still hope or expect a miraculous recovery. Our experience with such people has been that they never really do well until they are able to comprehend, and therefore deal with, the true meaning of renal failure.

The importance of family support toward patient well-being cannot be overemphasized. Recognizing the dependence the dialysis patient may feel, the enormous number of physical complications that may occur, the psychological stresses of an altered mode of life, the possible reversal of the normal husband-wife relationship, and the economic hardships which may be inflicted either temporarily or permanently, one can appreciate the importance of a mature understanding and supportive home environment. Unfortunately, a number of our patients and their families have been unable to make necessary adjustments in their home situations and have inflicted unnecessary emotional and physical trauma upon themselves.

Occasionally, patients experiencing personal problems are unable to acknowledge the cause and source of the problems, and rather than suffer the consequences of self-examination they look elsewhere for answers. A refusal to face reality is difficult to deal with, and despite intensive staff effort, results with patients who act thus remain unsatisfactory.

The intellectual capacity of patients is probably of some importance in relation to well-being, although the significance of intelligence as an isolated factor remains somewhat obscured by other more vital considerations. In studies performed several years ago in patients undergoing home dialysis, we found that patients whose IQ's were low but whose spouses IQ's were high did as well as patients whose IQ's were high, whether their spouses' IQ's were high or low.

In selecting children for maintenance dialysis, the parents as well as the child must be evaluated. A proper home environment is critical and understanding parents are essential. It is most important for children to resume their normal social activities as soon as possible, including school and play. We have seen well-meaning but overprotective parents impede the rehabilitation of their children by restricting their activities excessively. It is our feeling that, when possible, children should be offered transplantation as the modality of choice, and that for those requiring dialysis for any protracted period of time, it best be done in an area of the hospital separated from acutely or even chronically ill patients.

While the care of the sick ideally should never be equated with cost, unfortunately this has been the case in the past in regard to maintenance dialysis. Despite recent advances and progress in the treatment of renal failure, as yet inadequate facilities are available throughout the nation to meet the need of providing treatment to all. In some areas, there has been inadequate provision to care for the indigent. Accordingly, patients are still being denied therapy because of their inability to pay for it. We hope that recent federal legislation will eliminate the financial considerations relating to patient care in maintenance dialysis.

Once it has been decided to embark upon maintenance dialysis as opposed to immediate or almost immediate transplantation, a decision must be made as to whether dialysis should be done at home or in the center. A number of factors enter into this decision-making process, and these are discussed in the chapter dealing with home dialysis. In general, it is probably best to remain flexible in considering the modality of dialysis to be used, and to be in a position to offer a patient dialysis either at home or in an out-of-hospital center, with the possibility of switching from one to the other if the need arises. Almost all physicians now agree that the stable maintenance dialysis patient should leave the hospital and that the hospital should be reserved for patients requiring stabilization, those with medical problems, patients undergoing dialysis in relation to transplantation, and lastly, patients whose conditions are being monitored for teaching and investigation.

CARE OF THE PATIENT

It is most desirable to select patients for maintenance hemodialysis prior to their actual need for therapy. When progressive renal deterioration occurs in patients who are under the care of physicians relating to or participating in chronic dialysis programs, timely dialysis generally follows. As chronic renal failure supervenes and the serum creatinine rises to 10 mg/100 ml and above, it is usually appropriate to plan for dialysis, although this is a somewhat subjective determination. Since every dialysis program intends to keep the patient well in a prophylactic sense, we believe that whenever patients begin to show signs of being unable to perform adequate business, social, or personal functions because of mounting azotemia, dialysis should be considered. It is clear that such complications of uremia as pericarditis, neuropathy, pruritus, and metastatic calcifications are considerably more difficult to correct than to prevent. Accordingly, it is wise to treat the patient soon rather than hazard these complications as a result of procrastination and delay.

Again, it is difficult at best to evaluate patients for dialysis or transplantation while they are overtly uremic, apprehensive, unfamiliar with the personnel responsible for their care, and ignorant of the factors relating to maintenance dialysis. Because already overtly uremic patients are often referred for dialysis, it becomes necessary to treat and to stabilize them before beginning any evaluation procedure.

Gaining access to the blood supply was discussed in detail in Chapter 3. Regardless of whether cannulas are inserted or internal fistulas are established, these procedures should be done well in advance of the initial dialysis. It is best to insert a cannula 1 to 3 weeks prior to utilization, permitting the resultant edema and extravasation of blood to resolve and the patient's extremity to heal. The extremity should be rested and immobilized temporarily. Cannula longevity and extremity use appear to be inversely correlated.

It is at least equally important to establish the fistula well in advance of its initial use. In fact some of our best results have occurred when fistulas have been established months before the initial dialysis, and an opportunity has been afforded for the fistula to mature, the vessels to enlarge, and the walls to thicken. Although the effect of one or more fistulas on cardiac performance has been questioned, we have seen no patients in whom cardiac embarrassment resulted. This is discussed in greater detail in Chapter 6.

In patients selected early, the initial dialyses are usually uncomplicated. This assumes, of course, that the patient has been introduced to dialysis gradually with a series of short, frequent dialyses rather than an initial lengthy, vigorous treatment in an effort to produce a rapid reversal of the uremic syndrome. Just as it is preferable to initiate dialysis before the patient develops overt uremic symptomatology, it is also preferable to return the patient gradually to a more normal biochemical and physiological state. For example, a relatively asymptomatic average-sized patient may receive 2 or 3 hours of dialysis during his initial treatment and 3 or 4 hours 1 or two days later. However, the length of dialysis is heavily dependent upon the dialyzer used. In most centers today, predetermined commercially prepared dialysate baths are used for start-up dialysis—a good program that rarely needs modifying. However, in centers where individual baths are still made, it may be desirable to add up to 1000 gm of glucose to increase the initial bath osmolality. When a dialyzer requiring a blood pump is used, the flow should be kept relatively low during the initial treatments.

When patients are sick at the initial dialysis or particularly in the face of full-blown uremia, complications are far more likely and considerably more caution must be exercised. Peritoneal dialysis may be employed to correct the uremia gradually; anticonvulsants are generally in order. If hemodialysis is initiated, it should be carried out as an acute procedure. The patient should be separated from the stable maintenance dialysis patients; additional glucose should be added to the bath; signs and symptoms of dysequilibrium (see Chap. 8) as well as alterations in the cardiovascular status should be suspected.

When possible, avoid giving blood transfusions and priming the dialyzer with banked blood, even during the initial dialysis. This is of course determined to a large degree by the patient's age, clinical status, and hematocrit level. In general, the younger and the more stable the patient, the less likely he is to need blood. When a blood prime is required, packed red cells resuspended in saline or albumin, if necessary, are preferable. In potential transplant recipients, thawed, frozen red cells are preferable. This subject is covered further in Chapter 5.

Once the initial introductory period is over and the patient is on his way to stabilization, the physician must determine the frequency and number of hours of dialysis required. Current accepted medical practice to which we strongly adhere is dialysis at least 3 times a week. In fact, in the presence of such complications as pericarditis or neuropathy, we have dialyzed patients 4 or even 5 times a week.

Some measure of the adequacy of dialysis helps determine the number of hours of dialysis an individual requires. Unfortunately, present laboratory measures are rather crude and less reliable than one would like. Therefore, any determination as to the length of dialysis is based together on clinical experience, theoretical considerations, and commonly accepted medical practice. The actual length of dialysis must depend on the dialyzer used. Most of our clinical dialyses have been performed utilizing our point of reference, the Travenol Ultra-Flo dialyzers. We have generally dialyzed patients for from 4 to 6 hours 3 times a week, depending on body size and clinical requirements. With very small people (less than 90 pounds), we have reduced dialysis time to 3-½ hours and occasionally in large men, we have had to extend dialysis time to 7 hours. Until recently the gradient between blood and bath fluid was considered a critical factor in determining dialysis efficiency. Accordingly, shorter more frequent dialyses were considered more valuable than longer less frequent dialyses. However, with increasing cognizance of the importance of larger molecules with significiantly longer transport times in the production of the uremic syndrome, the importance of the gradient as relates to the efficiency of dialysis may diminish. This must be tempered, however, by our earlier experience when dialysis performed once or twice each week for many hours achieved poorer results. The final answer probably lies somewhere in the middle, with the gradient for smaller molecules such as urea and creatinine being relatively unimportant and the gradient for larger—and as yet unidentified—molecules having considerable importance. All available scientific information concerning objective criteria for the preference and requirement of dialysis at least 3 times a week is covered in the concluding paragraphs of Chapter 8.

Ongoing or follow-up care in patients undergoing maintenance dialysis usually depends on the individual and his needs. In general, the more reliable the patient, the less intensive his follow-up care must be. When patients have completed home training and embarked upon home dialysis, we usually see them on a monthly basis in an out-patient clinic. If the patient does well after approximately 6 months at home, we decrease the frequency of his routine visits to the center, first to every other month and then to every third month. We have seen patients on a semi-annual and even annual basis, but this should be reserved for selected patients.

By the nature of the selection process, patients undergoing dialysis at home have identified themselves as being more reliable and more capable of participating in their own care than patients receiving treatment in a center. Accordingly, they should require less medical intervention. On the other hand, patients who are dialyzed in a center, whether it be in-hospital or out-of-hospital, are seen by a physician during each visit. We recognize that not all patients treated in a center require daily physician supervision, but considering the population groups we deal with, anything less would seriously jeopardize too many of our patients. One disconcerting concern during the early days of out-of-hospital center dialysis was the anticipated need for hospital back-up, originally estimated at approximately 10 percent [6]. Since the home patients are by consensus more reliable and better motivated than the in-center patients, the back-up rate for the latter group might be even higher. For this reason we have considered the physician's visit during each dialysis critically valuable. The rate of hospital back-up for our out-of-hospital center patients consistently runs between 2 and 3 percent as compared to an 8 percent back-up rate for our home patients.

Early in our experience we obtained frequent laboratory studies. As our experience has increased, we have performed these studies less frequently and now obtain routine blood chemistries—including urea nitrogen, creatinine, calcium, phosphorus, alkaline phosphatase, bilirubin, uric acid, sodium, potassium, chloride, carbon dioxide content, and albumin and serum transaminases—every 2 months prior to dialysis in center patients and once every clinic visit for home patients. For the past 2 years, we have routinely screened patients every 3 months for Australia antigen. Hematocrit levels are routinely obtained during clinic visits for home patients and at least once each week for center patients. Electrocardiograms and chest x-rays are taken at 6- or 12-month intervals on a regular basis depending on the patient's clinical status. Radiographic bone studies and measurement of nerve conduction velocity are also obtained at 6-month intervals. These studies are discussed in detail in the chapters dealing with osteodystrophy and neurologic consequences.

Aside from those included in regular dialysis treatment, certain medications are necessary for continued patient well-being. Since phosphorus tends to accumulate resulting in hyperparathyroidism and osteodystrophy (discussed elsewhere), all patients under our care receive phosphate-binding gels. The form and type of drug administered are not critically important, and we have encountered no problems using preparations containing magnesium in out-patients. It is important, however, to monitor the serum phosphorus (and serum magnesium in those ingesting Mg^{++}-containing gels) and adjust the dosage according to individual patient need. We have usually prescribed 3 to 4 gm/day in divided doses, postprandially, but have increased this to from 12 to 15 gm/day when the need has arisen. It is more important for the patient to find a preparation he can tolerate than to take the most potent phosphate binder.

Because water-soluble vitamins are dialysable, we routinely administer multivitamins including folic acid to our patients, recognizing that most receive adequate vitamin replacement through their daily diet. We also routinely administer iron in the form of ferrous sulfate.

Some of our patients receive androgenic stimulation to foster erythropoiesis. Some women object because of potential hirsutism. We administer both oral and parenteral preparations, favoring the former as the initial choice because of ease of administration. We usually start with 20 mg/day of Halotestin (fluoxymesterone) increasing this to 40 mg/day or switching to an intramuscular preparation if necessary. Side effects necessitating discontinuance of the drug have been uncommon in our experience. However, several months of therapy may be required before any effect is seen, and not all patients respond. This subject is covered in more detail in Chapter 6. When side effects are seen a temporary reduction in drug dosage with a a subsequent return to previous levels may prove beneficial.

The potential disadvantages of blood transfusion in maintenance dialysis patients—the threat of hepatitis, the potential sensitization of those awaiting transplantation, and the depressive effect upon erythropoiesis all represent relative contraindications—are well known. Accordingly, we resist infusing red cells whenever possible, and symptomatic anemia is the sole indication for transfusion. In a group of patients followed over 36 months, the transfusion requirement was 0.23 units per patient per month. This figure includes 2 patients with massive gastrointestinal hemorrhage who required more than 75 units of blood each. After androgenic stimulation, the transfusion requirement dropped to 0.14 units per patient per month. More than half of our patients dialyzed 1 year or longer have, in fact, never required transfusion. The determination of symptomatic anemia is somewhat subjective and we have found that new house staff and younger physicians tend to transfuse earlier and more often, perhaps reflecting their apprehension. Supporting this somewhat is the fact that center patients have received more blood than home dialysis patients. When transfusing electively it is of value to infuse the freshest red cells available; cells more than several days old are of questionable value. There seems to be little indication for the elective use of whole blood.

Many patients have hypertension at the onset of dialysis treatment, which frequently responds readily to adequate dialysis and hyponatremic dehydration. In our experience, blood pressure falls toward normal after only a brief period of hemodialysis in more than 75 percent of patients. An additional 15 to 20 percent of patients require a more prolonged course of hemodialysis before blood pressure control and stabilization can be expected. Again, the mechanism invoked is hyponatremic dehydration. In a very few patients, blood pressure control is extremely difficult to achieve solely with dialysis. In some, a malignant picture develops accompanied by weight loss, heart failure, and progressive deterioration. While some of these patients may respond to drug therapy, including propranolol, most often we must resort to bilateral nephrectomy, which usually cures the hypertension. This subject is covered in detail in Chapter 5.

The blood pressure reading following bilateral nephrectomy may still depend upon the patient's state of hydration and may vary to the degree that intravascular volume is altered. However, even when the anephric patient is overhydrated and his blood pressure elevated, the malignant nature of the disease is usually no longer evident.

No phase of care relating to maintenance dialysis requires more time or patient effort than that which goes into the preparation and understanding of the diet. Most patients must make a substantial readjustment from previous habits. Frequently, during the progression of renal failure, salt loading has been encouraged; now a diametric change is required. Because the dietary constraints imposed by maintenance dialysis and chronic renal failure are long lasting, intelligent nutritional planning on the part of the staff and cooperation and comprehension on the part of the patient are necessary. It makes little sense to plan a diet not in keeping with a patient's eating habits.

Our patients are instructed to follow diets containing from as little as 500 mg of sodium and 2500 mg of potassium daily to as much as 4 gm of sodium and 3 gm of potassium. We encourage a rigid approach in those who tend toward hypertension, while we are more flexible with others. Since thirst generally relates to sodium intake, we have had to impose absolute fluid limitation in some patients who were either overhydrated or who had cardiac or hypertensive problems. Frequently, the water content of food must be reviewed. We normally do not limit protein; rather, we allow as much protein as possible within the limitations imposed by electrolyte restriction. If necessary, the length of dialysis is increased.

During dietary planning it is essential that the patient and dietician meet several times. Almost invariably the patient forgets or becomes confused during their initial meeting. Moreover, when the patient is not personally involved in preparing his meals, it is important to communicate with the individual bearing this responsibility. It is also valuable for the dietician to meet with the patient on a continuing basis, perhaps at intervals of 6 to 12 months.

Many patients are unaware of the large number of low-sodium foods available. This should be reviewed with them and they should be told where they can buy these foods. Several inexpensive handbooks that have been of great help to many patients list the composition of foods.

Once a patient has become stabilized on maintenance dialysis, concerted efforts should be made to enable him to resume his previous role in society. In situations in which the patient has not had to abandon work because of illness, this may not prove difficult, and the best results are often achieved in this group. Patients who have been forced to abandon work because of protracted illness find resuming normal activities more difficult. Both physical and vocational rehabilitative efforts may be required. With adequate dialysis and persistent physical therapy, several patients who were initially unable to walk as a result of severe peripheral neuropathy have strengthened their muscles sufficiently to walk again despite the lack of improvement in nerve function. It is vitally important to mobilize patients who have been bed fast as early as possible—the physical and emotional advantages of this are obvious. With this in mind, prolonged peritoneal dialysis seems undesirable and an early transfer to the artificial kidney prudent.

Some patients regard a return to work as an unnecessary meaningless exercise in futility. As a result of all the consequences of chronic renal failure, they sink into a deep depression from which they are unable to see any advantages to employment and are content to merely exist, resigned to the fact that there is no better life ahead for them. In this area and with these people a great deal of family, social worker, and psychiatric support must be provided. With understanding and adequate medical support, these patients may also respond in a positive manner and ultimately be rehabilitated.

REFERENCES

1. Murray, J.S., Tu, W.H., Albers, J.B., et al: A community hemodialysis center for the treatment of chronic uremia. Trans Am Soc Artif Intern Organs 8:315, 1962.

2. Subcommittee Report: Australian National Dialysis and Renal Transplantation Survey. Lancet 1:744, 1970.
3. Ghantous, W.N., Bailey, G.L., Zschaeck, D., et al: Long-term hemodialysis in the elderly. Trans Am Soc Artif Intern Organs 17:125, 1971.
4. Fine, R.N., Korsch, B.M., Grushkin, C.M., et al: Hemodialysis in children. Am J. Dis Child 119:498, 1972.
5. Chazan, J.I., Rees, S.B., Balodimos, M.C., et al: Dialysis in diabetics. JAMA 209:2026, 1969.
6. Pendras, J.P., and Pollard, T.L.: Eight years experience with a community dialysis center: The Northwest Kidney Center. Trans Am Soc Artif Intern Organs 16:77, 1970.

5

The Cardiovascular System

CARDIOVASCULAR STATUS IN CHRONIC RENAL FAILURE

In order to appreciate both the beneficial and possibly deleterious effects of hemodialysis on the cardiovascular system, it is necessary to consider all contributing factors. The basic abnormality is an increase in extracellular volume secondary to retention of sodium and water. This increase in volume is not only important in overloading the vascular system but also results in hypertension which in turn creates an increased work load on the heart, eventually leading to impairment of myocardial function.

Presystolic and/or protodiastolic gallop rhythms are commonly observed in uremic patients. Although these have been called "kidney gallops," [1] they are likely similar in origin to gallops heard in other types of heart disease. Cardiac catheterization studies in patients with uremia and fluid overload have yielded conflicting results. Pulmonary arterial pressure and right heart pressure have been demonstrated to be greater in uremic than in nonuremic patients [2,3], but not consistently so [4], and pressures in uremic patients are not as great as in patients with congestive heart failure from other causes [5]. It is generally assumed that pulmonary edema in the uremic patient is due to fluid overload or left ventricular failure, however, in the study by Gibson [5], observations in 7 uremic patients with acute pulmonary edema revealed that the pulmonary artery pressure was *lower* than that observed in patients with pulmonary edema due to mitral stenosis or left ventricular failure. Similar findings by Mostert et al [2] support the interpretation that there is a component of increased pulmonary capillary permeability in renal failure. The clinical importance of increased pulmonary capillary permeability in producing the so-called uremic lung remains to be elucidated. In our experience most cases of uremic lung result from simple fluid overload and respond to usual treatment of pulmonary edema. Nevertheless, we treat most affected individuals with dialysis (and ultrafiltration) so that it is difficult to rule out in the individual patient a correction of an underlying abnormal pulmonary vascular permeability by dialysis of the uremia per se.

Factors other than increased extracellular volume and hypertension contributing to altered function of the myocardium are severe anemia and biochemical derangements such as hyperkalemia, hypocalcemia, hypermagnesemia and acidosis—all of which may effect the conduction system, general cardiac irritability, and/or myocardial contractility. The myocardium has probably been affected by hypertension as well as arteriosclerotic coronary artery disease, which is more likely to occur in the uremic patient because of the hypertension and the following considerations:

Uremic hyperlipidemia has been described by Bagdade and his coworkers [6]. These investigators demonstrated increased triglyceride, decreased lipoprotein lipase, and increased immunoreactive insulin in non-nephrotic uremic patients. The authors speculated that this was due to increased hepatic synthesis of triglyceride-rich lipoprotein and to decreased removal of triglyceride as reflected by the low lipase. In our patient population we have also found an increase in serum triglycerides more frequently than would be expected in a normal population. Lipid electrophoresis most commonly revealed type IV hyperlipidemia. After beginning hemodialysis the incidence increased even further despite correction of previously deranged carbohydrate metabolism. Type IV hyperlipidemia is associated with an increased incidence of arteriosclerotic heart disease, although to a lesser extent than are types II or III hyperlipidemia [7]. These findings and the subject of hyperlipidemia are discussed in more detail in Chapter 9.

Another risk factor in uremia is the presence of advanced vascular coronary artery calcification related to hyperparathyroidism. Metastatic calcification involving the coronary arteries has been well documented in uremic patients [8-11] and may lead to myocardial fibrosis with congestive heart failure. In addition to calcification of the coronary arteries, there may be myocardial calcification [12,13], which is particularly ominous when it involves the conduction system. Terman et al [14] described 6 patients with moderate to severe metastatic calcification of the myocardium. First degree heart block was found in 5, atrioventricular conduction delay in 5, and complete heart block in 2. Two patients died suddenly and 2 suffered intractable congestive heart failure. We can attribute several sudden deaths in our program to myocardial or coronary arterial calcification and have noted 2 further patients in whom severe calcification of the aortic valves was felt to be associated with the presence of severe secondary hyperparathyroidism.

Most patients with renal insufficiency have had low-protein diets prescribed for varying periods of time. Potential protein deficiency may be accentuated by chronic anorexia and nausea and vomiting. Vitamin deficiency may likewise result unless vitamin supplementation is given. Bailey, Hampers, and Merrill [15] reported 5 patients with a peculiar cardiomyopathy that responded to hemodialysis. Its exact cause was not delineated, although possible causes were: hypoproteinemia, soluble B-vitamin deficiency, hypertensive or arteriosclerotic cardiovascular disease, and/or the presence of an unidentified uremic toxin adversely affecting myocardial function. Deterioration in cardiac function correlated with initiation of the diet and with declining renal function. These patients improved with hemodialysis and liberalization of diet with increased protein. Thus the authors felt that this causally incriminated either dietary deficiency or the presence of some uremic toxic substance; however, hypertension was difficult to rule out as a major factor. In summary, increased serum triglycerides (and resultant atherosclerosis), vascular calcification, hypertension, anemia, and nutritional, metabolic, and biochemical disturbances may all combine to various degrees to adversely affect the myocardium in the patient on chronic hemodialysis who is already prone to fluid overload because of limited excretory ability.

In addition to myocardial disturbances, uremic patients often have involvement of the endocardium (i.e., valvular disease) and pericardium. Many uremic patients have systolic ejection murmurs (the significance of which is difficult to determine) that may be quite harsh and loud and are characteristically of short duration in early to midsystole. We feel that they are usually hemic or flow murmurs related to the severe anemia. Although diastolic murmurs are considered indicative of organic disease, such murmurs have been described in patients with chronic renal failure and disappear with adequate hemodialysis [16] or have been shown to occur in the absence of organic findings at postmortem examination [17]. Valvular calcification due to hyperparathyroidism, previously mentioned, may follow or accentuate preexisting valvular disease. Murmurs resulting from endocarditis must be distinguished from the benign murmur referred to above. Impaired immunologic capabilities render these patients more prone to systemic infections. Septicemia and septic pulmonary embolization [18-21], as well as bacterial endarteritis [22], have been well-documented in patients with arteriovenous shunts and fistulas—prime sites for entrance of bacteria into the circulation. In the original report of the arteriovenous fistula by Brescia and his co-workers [23], a patient is described who developed valvular incompetence following fistula insertion. Goodman et al [24] have reported 2 cases of bacterial endocarditis in chronic hemodialysis patients, and other reports have followed [25-27]. We have had at least 4 patients with sepsis felt to be related to bacterial endocarditis. Two of these patients subsequently developed intractable congestive heart failure because of aortic insufficiency and underwent prosthetic valvular replacement. Patients with suspected or proven bacterial endocarditis should be treated with intravenous antibiotics for at least 6 weeks. If valvular incompetence develops and interferes with myocardial function, surgical repair should be considered. In most cases, the problem is not clear-cut—septicemia occurs in patients with arteriovenous fistulas or shunts which may or may not appear infected, and no changes are reflected in the cardiac examination. We have assumed these cases are endarteritis and have modified the treatment regimen by prescribing intravenous antibiotics for 10 days to 2 weeks and then maintaining oral antibiotics for another 4 to 5 weeks. On three occasions we have ligated arteriovenous fistulas because of recurring septicemia; each time, the problem resolved. The differential with endocarditis is difficult, especially since uremic patients seem to have a propensity for developing bacterial endocarditis. Causing scarring of the valves, endocarditis might be a contributing factor to poor cardiac performance and must be considered in patients with congestive heart failure not responding to hemodialysis.

Pericarditis is common in the uremic patient and will be discussed in detail subsequently. Occasionally uremic patients develop cardiac tamponade secondary to hemorrhagic pericardial effusion [28-30]. Constrictive pericarditis, heretofore almost unheard of in uremia, has now been described [31-33] as chronic hemodialysis patients are kept alive for longer periods of time. This entity must also be considered in the differential diagnosis of heart failure in patients maintained with the artificial kidney.

We have recently demonstrated an abnormal baroreceptor reflex sensitivity in uremic patients [34]. This blunted baroreceptor reflex has also been described in hypertensive patients [35] and in patients with primary cardiovascular disease [36]. In Figure 1 are shown the

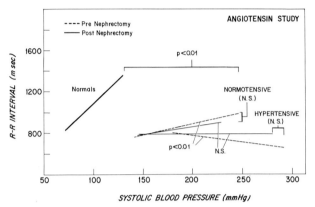

Fig. 1. Slopes of mean linear regressions developed by measuring the R-R interval (1/pulse) with elevation of systolic blood pressure by intravenous angiotensin. Hypertensive uremic patients had mean slope significantly lower than normotensive uremic patients. Difference was less following bilateral nephrectomy with its lowering of blood pressure. Before and after nephrectomy, slopes in hypertensive and normotensive uremic patients were all significantly less than those of normal controls.

slopes of the linear regressions of the pulse response to elevation of blood pressure demonstrated in normal controls and normotensive and hypertensive uremic patients, both before and after bilateral nephrectomy. All uremic patients, regardless of the presence of hypertension, with or without nephrectomy, showed a blunted baroreceptor response. That is, they did not develop the bradycardia one would expect with a given *increase* in blood pressure. More importantly, uremic patients did not show the expected tachycardia with *lowering* of the blood pressure. This is illustrated in Figure 2, which shows the results of administration of amyl nitrite to uremic patients and controls. These studies demonstrate an impaired response in uremic patients, probably on the basis of an abnormal baroreceptor mechanism. This conclusion is supported by studies on the cardiovascular response to Valsalva maneuver [3,37], upright posture [38,39], and to other drugs [40,41]. It is theorized that the abnormal baroreceptor mechanism is due to neuropathy of the autonomic nervous system with contributions by preexisting hypertension, myocardial disease, and chronic anemia.

The pulmonary system is frequently involved in patients with chronic renal failure. This involvement may consist of pleuritis, pleural effusion, pulmonary edema, or altered pulmonary vascular permeability

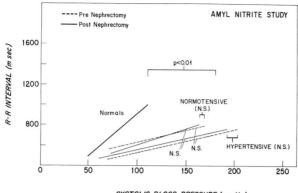

Fig. 2. Slopes of mean linear regressions developed by plotting the R-R interval (1/pulse) with systolic blood pressure lowered by amyl nitrite inhalation. Before and after bilateral nephrectomy, normotensive and hypertensive uremic patients had mean slopes significantly lower than those of normal controls.

as explained earlier. The relationship of uremia to pleuritis with chest pain and pleural friction rub has been discussed by Nidus et al [42]. We agree with their reported incidence of approximately 15 percent. All or any of these pulmonary complications may compromise óxygen exchange and provide an additional detrimental effect on the heart. Hemodialysis usually resolves the problem of fluid overload and may in addition reverse the suspected abnormal pulmonary vascular permeability. Pleuritis often resolves promptly; however, plural effusions resolve several weeks later. Thoracocentesis should be considered when pleural effusions may compromise pulmonary function. This should be performed on a *nondialysis* day, however, and regional heparinization used in the following hemodialysis.

Uremic patients frequently require bed rest for prolonged periods and might predictably be prime candidates for recurrent pulmonary emboli. This has not been the case. Pulmonary embolization is extremely unusual in a uremic or dialysis population. It is theorized that decreased viscosity with anemia and a somewhat decreased clotting time (secondary to poor platelet adhesion and decrease in platelet factor 3) explain the rarely documented occurrence of pulmonary emboli in this group.

The effects of large traumatically induced arteriovenous fistulas on cardiac function have been studied extensively [43-45], and it has been concluded that they may lead to the development of frank congestive heart failure. With the widespread use of shunts and fistulas for chronic hemodialysis, further evaluation of the effect of shunts on myocardial function has been carried out. Dotremont et al [46] found that occlusion of the arteriovenous fistula elicited a slight decrease in heart rate and an increase in arterial pressure and total peripheral resistance. However, the change in the cardiac output in the majority of patients was not different from that of the control group. Heidland et al [47] and Franz et al [48] similarly found no or only minor change in cardiac output with compression of the AV fistulas. With exercise, but not at rest, Payne et al [49] and Dotremont demonstrated significantly increased cardiac output in patients with fistulas as compared to controls. Other investigators [50-54], however, have suggested there is an increased cardiac output at rest, having found a significant reduction in cardiac output with occlusion of AV fistulas. The causal relationship between this increased cardiac output and subsequent congestive heart failure or pulmonary edema has not been so well demonstrated. Johnson and Blythe found no clinical evidence of cardiomegaly or congestive heart failure, Hanson et al [55] observed no cardiac embarrassment in 15 patients with AV fistulas, and Hurwich [56] found similar flows in shunts and fistulas and felt they were not large enough to create a serious burden on the heart. Payne et al concluded that little hemodynamic deterioration occurred with AV fistulas and instances of congestive heart failure were more likely due to fluid overload and underdialysis. McMillan et al [57] and Ahern and Maher [58], however, have reported what appears to be a cause-effect relationship between large AV fistulas in the extremities and intractable congestive heart failure. It seems likely that with increasing numbers of patients being treated with the artificial kidney and medical criteria for selection being liberalized, some of these patients might have borderline cardiac function and a slight increase in cardiac demand may make the critical difference. Therefore, fistulas may in some patients be enough to tip the balance toward heart failure. In our own experience with more than 600 patients, we have never felt it necessary to band or remove an access in order to control congestive heart failure. In all instances, heart failure has been adequately managed with control of other contributing factors.

Cardiac output or cardiac index in uremic patients has been found to be increased in most reports [2-4,59,62], while others have described normal findings [37,63,65] or great variability [66]. All of the factors discussed in the preceding section may have a mixed effect on cardiac output—that is, anemia, compromised pulmonary function, sepsis, fever, and arteriovenous shunts and fistulas may *increase* cardiac output; other factors—such as increased extracellular volume, decreased myocardial contractility, arrhythmias, pericardial disease with effusions, incompetent valves, blunted baroreceptor responses and increased total peripheral resistance—may all tend to *decrease* cardiac output. All of these factors potentially contribute to myocardial failure and each must be considered in evaluating a patient's particular cardiovascular picture.

THE EFFECT OF HEMODIALYSIS ON THE CARDIOVASCULAR SYSTEM

The major effect of hemodialysis on the cardiovascular system is established through reducing intravascular fluid volume, interstitial fluid, and finally intracellular fluid. The shift of fluid from the intracellular space to extracellular space may be slower than the rate of water removal by the dialyzer. Thus, despite the fact that other fluid compartments (interstitial and intracellular) may still be hypervolemic, the immediate effect is vascular volume depletion.

During hemodialysis cardiac output has been variably shown to increase or remain unchanged, depending on the presence of circulatory congestion, volume depletion, or other factors. DelGreco et al [64,66] demonstrated the importance of preexisting circulatory congestion on the effect of hemodialysis on cardiac output. Cardiac output improved with hemodialysis in a greater percentage of patients with circulatory congestion than in patients without congestive features. Hampers and co-workers [37] likewise demonstrated the importance of volume status in determining the effect of hemodialysis on cardiac output. They found no consistent change in cardiac output after hemodialysis if plasma volume was kept constant. Intradialysis studies by Goss et al [2] revealed a decrease in cardiac index during the procedure, while use of the ballistocardiogram in evaluating cardiac output by Henderson and associates [65] demonstrated no change in cardiac output during the procedure. These studies were concerned with the acute effects of the dialysis procedure. Patients stabilized on hemodialysis have long-term improvement in myocardial function as indicated by an overall increase in cardiac output [67]. Total peripheral resistance has been found to be increased in approximately 50 percent of patients with chronic renal failure [3,4,66], and this usually correlates with the presence of hypertension [61,62]. During dialysis, peripheral resistance increases [2,37,66] probably in response to contraction of plasma volume.

In patients with a precarious cardiovascular status, too rapid reduction in intravascular fluid may have disastrous results. To avoid such an effect, the hemodialyzer and lines should be filled with normal saline, plasma, or some suitable colloid, which is returned to the patient at the same rate blood is removed, thereby maintaining constant volume. Because of the high incidence of sensitization to transplantation antigens, problems with hepatitis, and expense, whole blood primes should be avoided. Since patients have an expanded extracellular volume between dialysis, it is possible to slowly bleed the patient into the dialyzing reservoir without volume for volume replacement with little consequence. This is a helpful procedure in reducing the total fluid compartment, but careful evaluation of the cardiovascular status of each patient at the time of such a procedure is obviously necessary.

Many factors affect fluid removal during hemodialysis. Variabilities within each dialysis system—such as configuration of the dialyzer, type of membrane, and surface area—determine the ultrafiltration characteristics. These factors can be further modified by increasing or decreasing outflow resistance, altering blood or dialysate flowrates, or by increasing or decreasing osmolality of the dialyzing fluid—principles discussed previously. Occasionally, a patient with a marked extracellular volume excess demonstrates unstable blood pressure with frequent hypotension, thereby making ultrafiltration difficult if not impossible. Kim et al [68] have suggested using a dextran prime to avoid such problems. The technique we have found most helpful, however, is metaraminol (200 mg in 500 cc of normal saline) given as a drip to maintain blood pressure during hemodialysis. This allows ultrafiltrative maneuvers to be carried out while maintaining blood pressure. However, postdialysis postural hypotension often occurs after the procedure. Such problems can be avoided by maintaining the patient in the supine position for 15 to 20 minutes and gradually elevating him to the upright position.

The removal of simple extracellular fluid may precede by days the removal of fluid from so-called third spaces, such as are found with pleural effusions, pericardial effusions, and ascites. These third space fluids should be essentially ignored when estimating volume replacement. Ultrafiltration and volume shifts by the dialyzer can dramatically affect extracellular and intravascular volume, thereby creating varied effects on the cardiovascular system. Careful evaluation of the individual patient before dialysis must be the basis for selecting the appropriate maneuver.

In addition to the effects of exsanguination and ultrafiltration, there is an added effect of the extracorporeal system per se on cardiovascular hemodynamics. This effect may be simply inapparent vascular volume reduction [68,69]; however, patients sometimes develop tachycardia, hypotension, or other symptoms of volume depletion despite the most exacting volume replacement. This occurs more frequently in small children, elderly patients with preexisting myocardial disease, and acute, postoperative patients—obviously the very patients in whom one desires to avoid wide swings in blood pressure. Important in this phenomenon are blood flow rate and total volume of blood in the extracorporeal circuit. Another frequent symptom, seen with a too rapid onset of hemodialysis, is aching low back pain. This can be reversed by slowing the blood flow rate. While the cause of this often excruciating back pain is unknown, it may be related to ischemia of the lower spine as dialysis proceeds or to the sudden infusion of a foreign substance (e.g., heparin or preservative material on dialysis membrane). Fortunately, it is rarely of clinical import and subsides after a few minutes of dialysis with a slowed blood flow rate.

More serious consequences of early rapid blood flow into the dialyzer are the precipitation of cardiac arrhythmias or angina pectoris or both. If cardiovascular instability is suspected, not only should the patient have milliliter for milliliter volume replacement, but dialysis should be initiated very slowly as well. Reduction of the dialyzing blood volume through use of small plate dialyzers, hollow fiber kidneys or smaller volume coil kidneys appears to help manage patients who seem to tolerate the initiation of dialysis poorly. One must carefully weigh the need for low volume and slow flow against other considerations such as the need for ultrafiltration and the minimum dialyzing surface required to control uremia. A delicate balance should be determined for each patient.

Patients with prior history of myocardial infarction, angina pectoris, arrhythmias, or cerebral insufficiency often tolerate dialysis better if hematocrit levels are maintained above 30 percent. These are and should be exceptions to the policy of not regularly transfusing patients on chronic dialysis. Routine digitalization in most dialysis patients with heart disease has not been found valuable; however, occasionally patients may benefit. In our own program we attempt to minimize the use of cardiovascular, antihypertensive, and antiarrhythmic drugs in patients undergoing hemodialysis. Such preparations, which may be necessary in the uremic patient prior to the institution of dialysis, can usually be discontinued as the patient is regulated with dialysis and ultrafiltration. If digitalis is necessary the drug of choice is Digoxin, which is most rapidly metabolized. Less than 3 percent of the drug has been found in dialysate fluid and therefore the effect of dialysis may for practical purposes be ignored [70]. While a number of formulas are available for the calculation of dosage, the usual dose in our dialysis population has been 0.125 mg every day or every other day. Since digitalis intoxication is particularly difficult to detect in uremic patients, it is frequently necessary (as it is in many nonuremic patients) to discontinue digitalis preparations in order to appreciate their toxic effects.

Obviously important in the patient receiving digitalis is the maintenance of a fairly stable serum potassium level. The effect of potassium in the uremic patient is, however, important whether digitalis is given or not. In 1953 Kohn and Kiley [71] demonstrated that some specific electrocardiographic changes in the terminally uremic patient were probably due to potassium and reverted with lowering of the serum potassium. Levine, Wapzer, and Merrill [72] described changes in the electrocardiogram similar to those seen in patients with pericarditis or myocardial infarction; this "current of injury" had been reversed with hemodialysis. The classical electrocardiographic changes of hyperkalemia so often seen in renal insufficiency have been well described and are valuable in following such patients [73,74]. DelGreco and Grumer [75] and Rubin et al [76] reviewed electrocardiograms of patients undergoing hemodialysis and also demonstrated not only S-T and T-wave changes but varied supraventricular and ventricular arrhythmias precipitated by the lowering of serum potassium. One must be careful in interpreting electrocardiograms during the hemodialysis procedure for, in addition to these "real" arrhythmias it has been shown that pseudoarrhythmias may appear secondary to action of the blood pump [77]. These usually present as ventricular or atrial parasystoles and can be detected because of regular periodicity and correlation in time with the hemodialysis pump. Whenever possible, the blood pump should be discontinued when an electrocardiogram is being obtained.

Serum potassium in patients on hemodialysis is affected by changes in general acid-base balance but more obviously by removal of potassium in the dialyzer. The appropriate potassium concentration in the dialysate bath has been the subject of much discussion. Investigators have altered the dialysate potassium to evaluate serum levels and the occurrence of arrhythmias. Johnson et al [78], Seedat [79], and Johny [80] found that three times a week hemodialysis with a 0 to 1 mEq/liter potassium bath concentration was sufficient to induce total body potassium depletion. Morgan et al [81] demonstrated that three times a week hemodialysis with a 1.5 mEq/liter potassium level did not cause depletion; however, one-half of these patients experienced *hypo*kalemia following hemodialysis and mild *hyper*kalemia before the subsequent hemodialysis. Our experience has been similar. Patients demonstrate serum potassium levels of 2 to 3 mEq/liter during or immediately follow-ing hemodialysis when the potassium bath concentration is 2 mEq/liter, but they have serum potassium values in the 4.5 to 6 mEq/liter range 36 to 48 hours following hemodialysis with a dietary potassium of 2 gm/day.

The effectiveness of hemodialysis in correcting dangerous acute hyperkalemia has been well documented. The electrocardiogram in Figure 3 is an example of such a case. This is the cardiogram of a 16-year-old chronic dialysis patient brought to the dialysis unit with low blood pressure, decreased mentation, rapid tachycardia, and a serum potassium level of 9.2 mEq/liter. The electrocardiogram reverted to normal accompanied by rapid clinical improvement during the hemodialysis procedure. One should be careful to lower the serum potassium cautiously, beginning with a dialysate-potassium concentra-tion of 3 to 4 mEq/liter and slowly lowering the bath concentration to 0 over a 2- to 4-hour period. In most instances hyperkalemia of this degree can be related to dietary misadventures.

The importance of the serum potassium in the para-operative period has been commented upon in the literature [82]. We routinely dialyze patients 12 to 24 hours prior to anticipated surgery using between 2 mEq/L and 0 potassium concentration in the dialysate. This generally allows the patient to finish dialysis with a serum potassium level of approximately 2.5 to 3.5 mEq/liter, and by the next morning (at the time of surgery) the serum potassium is generally 3.5 to 4.5 mEq/liter. We do not operate if the potassium level is greater than 5.0 mEq/liter at the time of surgery. This program must be modified in the dialysis patient on a digitalis preparation. Utilizing such a policy, episodes of intraoperative arrhythmia have been minimized. We have had experi-ence with more than 400 major surgical procedures in our dialysis population and consider these patients good candidates, although post-operative morbidity is slightly higher than in nondialysis patients. In addition to controlling serum potassium, we adjust the hematocrit to a level to 25 vol% or above. One must be careful not to dehydrate the patient too severely before surgery since this may result in intra-operative difficulties with early hypotension. The anesthesiology department must be aware of the limited excretory capacity of certain drugs in this group of patients in avoiding intoxications. Careful pre-and post-operative management is essential if early postoperative dialysis under regional heparinization is to be used. Occasionally daily dialysis is required in the immediate postoperative period in order to control hypercatabolism, but this must be individualized. Certainly surgery should *not* be withheld from a dialysis patient simply because he is a dialysis patient if the indications for operation are present.

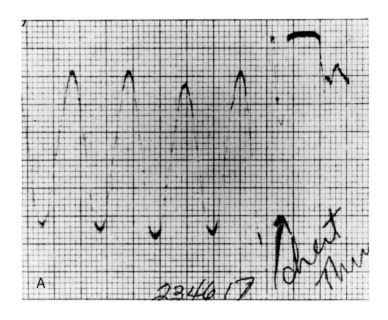

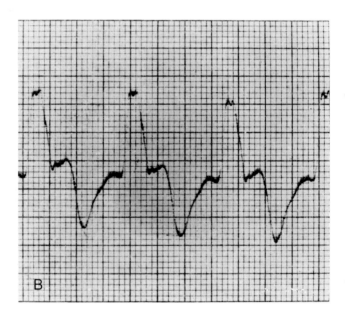

Fig. 3. Serial electrocardiograms of 16-year-old chronic dialysis patient who presented with hypotension, tachyrhythmia, and a serum potassium concentration of 9.2 mEq/L after dietary indiscretion. First strip (A) taken immediately after admission. Subsequent evolution (B)–(D), occurred after the patient was

90

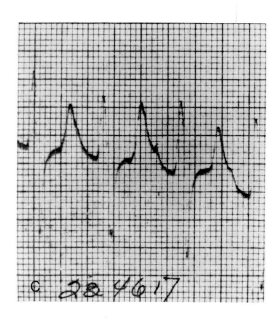

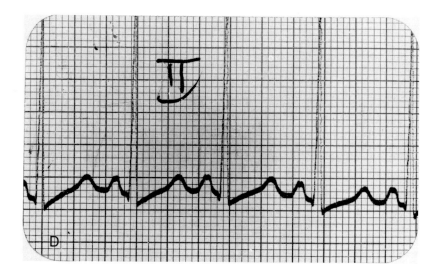

dialyzed against dialysis baths with progressively lower potassium levels. Reversion of EKG changes paralleled improvement in hypotension and other clinical symptoms.

PERICARDIAL DISEASE

Uremic pericarditis is a common complication of uremia occurring in approximately 30 to 50 percent of patients with terminal renal failure [83-85]. This estimate, which is based on the clinical diagnosis of pericarditis, is supported by postmortem studies reporting the incidence of a fibrinous pericardium [86-87]. The most definitive and often the only premortem evidence of pericarditis is a pericardial friction rub, often heard only in systole, but usually distinguishable from systolic murmurs by its typical quality. A multicomponent rub clearly makes the diagnosis easier. It may be loud and heard over the entire pericardium but frequently is localized and may be missed if it is not searched for carefully. Pericardial rubs in uremic patients are often transient— they may be heard in the morning, disappear late in the afternoon, and reappear in the evening or the next day. In our experience, the second most common sign of pericarditis is fever, frequently low grade and usually following the onset of the friction rub. The presence of chest pain may be quite variable in quality but is usually substernal and classically is relieved by sitting up or leaning forward. Any chest pain in a uremic patient should alert one to the possibility of pericarditis. On occasion, the typical electrocardiographic findings of ST elevation are present, but in practice we rarely have found this to be of value. The chest roentgenogram in early pericarditis is likewise unrevealing except to reassure the examiner that there is no massive accumulation of fluid. An isolated left pleural effusion is frequently seen and should alert one to the possibility of pericardial disease.

Prior to the availability of hemodialysis, pericarditis was felt to be a sign of impending death [83]. It remains an important sign even now, indicating the need for hemodialysis. In one of the first postmortem studies of uremic patients, Bright [88] noted the occurrence of pericarditis with inflammation of other serosal surfaces, suggesting a general involvement secondary to the disease. Although viral or bacterial infection [86,90] and concomitant myocarditis [91,92] may be responsible for occasional cases of pericarditis, most feel that the pericardial inflammation is caused by a metabolic-chemical response secondary to an accumulated uremic product. The rapid disappearance of pericarditis with the initiation of hemodialysis strongly supports this contention. Resolution of the pericardial rub generally parallels overall improvement in the patient on hemodialysis. Exceptions to this rule include patients with systemic lupus erythematosis or scleroderma. Pericarditis may recur or appear for the first time weeks or months after the initiation of hemodialysis. We feel that pericarditis in patients on dialysis is usually associated with some concurrent stress such as surgery, trauma, or generalized infection. When a pericardial friction rub appears in a chronically dialyzed patient without one of these factors, it may well be due to viral pericarditis although such a diagnosis has been difficult to substantiate. Indeed, the appearance of pericarditis without an obvious cause in patients on maintenance dialysis should be considered a sign of inadequate dialysis until proven otherwise. We consider the occurrence of a pericardial rub (regardless of its cause) as indication for either the initiation of dialysis or (in those already being treated with dialysis) an increase in the frequency of dialysis.

Obviously, patients being initiated on hemodialysis should be evaluated carefully by the physician prior to each dialysis for a pericardial rub. If present, dialysis should be performed with regional heparinization until the rub has disappeared for at least two or three dialyses. One must be aware of the possibility of heparin rebound [93] and its effect on patients with pericarditis. To reduce the effects of late heparinization, we frequently administer protimine (approximately 50 percent of the total heparin dose) at the close of regional heparinization. Corticosteroids have been reported to hasten the resolution of uremic pericardial effusion [90]. It is our impression, however, that this treatment does *not* affect the disappearance of the rub nor does it reduce the liklihood of later effusion or constrictive pericarditis.

Although hemorrhagic pericardial effusions have been reported in nondialyzed uremic patients [28,92,94-96], the incidence of this complication is increased by the use of heparin for hemodialysis [30]. There is early granulation tissue between the two inflamed pericardial layers [96] and with normal myocardial movement and abrasion of these surfaces, bloody pericardial effusion is likely to result, particularly in the presence of heparin. Indeed, pericardial effusions have been reported to be uniformly bloody [28-30,97,98], and in our experience hematocrit levels of the effusions approach that of the peripheral blood. It may be difficult to determine whether the ventricular or atrial chambers have been entered during pericardiocentesis. The pericardial fluid, however, is usually darker than venous blood and if it clots, as it sometimes does, the serum is usually red with hemolyzed blood. Injection of radiocontrast material or indocyanine green [99] may help determine the location of the pericardiocentesis needle.

A frequent sign of early accumulation of fluid is the disappearance of a previously loud friction rub. Since one expects the pericardial rub to disappear with hemodialysis, the differential diagnosis may be difficult. Early or moderate fluid accumulation without compromise of cardiac function may be especially difficult to detect. Most helpful at this point is the chest x-ray and the careful evaluation of a changing cardiac silhouette. If the presence of fluid is still questioned, a number of diagnostic procedures are available. Currently, the simplest and most noninvasive method is the echocardiogram or ultrasound study, [100-102] which we have found very reliable. Carbon dioxide contrast studies can be performed with a CO_2 source and a lateral decubitus chest film [103,104]. More sophisticated but probably no more reliable techniques are intracardiac angiography and a radioisotope scan [107].

In patients with pericardial effusions that are not hemodynamically significant, we continue hemodialysis with regional heparinization and close clinical observation. We reserve pericardiocentesis for patients with clinical symptoms of cardiac tamponade. In the patient with gross fluid overload, ultrafiltration may occasionally be important in reducing pericardial fluid. More often, however, the resolution of pericardial fluid is related to improvement in clotting properties and overall reduction of the pericardial inflammation such as occurs with the correction of the uremic state.

A small percentage of patients with mild to moderate pericardial effusions later develop pericardial tamponade despite conservative attempts to reabsorb the effusion. The literature is replete with case reports of cardiac tamponade due to uremic pericarditis [28-30,84, 85,97,98]. We estimate that this complication occurs in less than 10 percent of our patients with pericardial effusions. The signs and symptoms of tamponade are well known and include an increase in the jugular venous pressure, a prominent hepatic jugular reflux, a "quiet" precordium with no palpable PMI, decreasing heart sounds, pulses paradoxicus of greater than 10mm Hg, and usually a large globular heart with oligemic-appearing lung fields. Occasionally, the electrocardiogram may show a decrease in voltage. With significant cardiac tamponade there is a decrease in the ventricular diastolic filling gradient and a decrease in cardiac output. This may be accentuated in the patient undergoing hemodialysis, being manifested as rapid and profound hypotension as the patient is placed on the extracorporeal circuit or with ultrafiltration efforts to reduce apparent excessive extracellular volume. In our experience, this is frequently seen before the occurrence of paradoxical pulse or the other usual signs of tamponade. Patients suspected of having significant effusion should be followed closely to insure that pericardiocentesis is carried out electively rather than as an emergency.

Pericardiocentesis is performed by the method described by Bailey et al [85] percutaneous utilizing a 14- to 16-gauge catheter through a 4th left intercostal space entry. After the catheter is advanced to the bottom of the pericardial sac, the patient can be rotated or moved to insure removal of maximal amounts of fluid. This method is used when the tamponade is large and the procedure can be performed easily without the need for EKG monitoring of the needle tip. If the amount of fluid is smaller, the preferred method is the use of a spinal needle with EKG monitoring through a subxyphoid approach. We have found the insertion of air into the pericardium in a ratio of 1 cc for every 2 cc of fluid removed to be beneficial in patients undergoing hemodialysis with heparinization (Fig. 4). This technique keeps the visceral and parietal layers of pericardium apart, thereby decreasing friction and further hemorrhage into the closed space. One must obviously be certain the needle is in the pericardial space before inserting

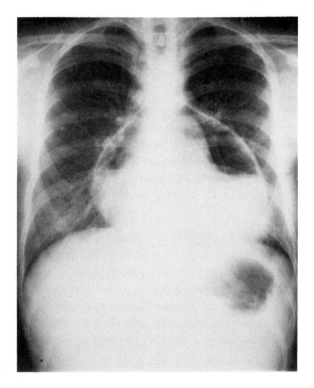

Fig. 4. Chest x-ray of 17-year-old girl on chronic dialysis following pericardiocentesis for hemorrhagic tamponade. Air was replaced 1 ml for every 2 ml of effusion removed. Air and the remaining bloody effusion resolved over the next 2 weeks with regional heparinization and increased dialysis frequency.

air. Most uremic patients with cardiac tamponade can be handled by this conservative approach (without surgery) along with increased dialysis time and regional heparinization. Some reports advocate pericardectomy when signs of tamponade recurr or continue [98] after a single pericardiocentesis. On the other hand, we frequently repeat pericardiocentesis 2 or 3 times before recommending surgery. With this approach in the past 5 years, we have had to perform pericardectomy for tamponade on only 3 occasions. When surgery is required the usual procedure is a subtotal pericardectomy or the creation of a sufficiently large pericardial "window" so that fibrous adhesions cannot subsequently seal the margins of the pericardium.

With increasing use of chronic hemodialysis and prolongation of life in more patients with acute pericarditis, constrictive pericarditis—a previously rare condition—has become more common. This was first reported in 1964 by Traeger et al [31] and Hager [29] and subsequently was documented in a number of reports [32,33,108-112]. The picture is one of decreasing cardiac output with signs as described for cardiac tamponade. However, it differs from tamponade in that a small heart is seen on chest x-ray and there is usually edema of the lower extremities and ascites due to the slow chronic obstruction of the venous return. Figure 5 illustrates the cardiac silhouette during the course of a patient with constrictive pericarditis who presented with symptoms of postural hypotension, edema, and neck vein engorgement. In another patient the diagnosis was suspected because of persistently low blood pressures on hemodialysis with increased extracellular volume and a small heart by x-ray examination.

The incidence of constrictive pericarditis is extremely low—we have seen only 2 cases. When constrictive pericarditis is suspected, the diagnosis should be substantiated by cardiac catheterization which classically reveals a decrease. in cardiac output and an increased right atrial pressure [109,110]. The treatment of choice for constrictive pericarditis is pericardectomy, which should be carried out at the earliest possible moment before the constriction interferes with adequate hemodialysis and further complicates the institution of corrective surgery.

HYPERTENSION

Hypertension is the most frequent cardiovascular complication of chronic renal failure. We estimate that over 80 percent of patients with renal failure requiring hemodialysis have blood pressure recordings in excess of 150/90, although many are asymptomatic. Other patients,

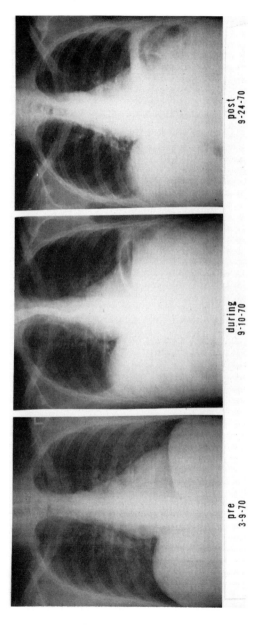

pre
3-9-70

during
9-10-70

post
9-24-70

Fig. 5. Serial chest x-rays of 46-year-old patient with pericardial effusion that resolved with regional heparinization and increased dialysis frequency. One year later he developed postural hypotension, mild ankle edema, and blood flow maintenance difficulty on dialysis because of hypotension. Cardiac catheterization revealed systolic arterial pressure 74/44 mm Hg [54], right atrial pressure 18 mm Hg [54 with Valsalva], right ventricular pressure 30/18 mm Hg, pulmonary artery pressure of 28/18 mm Hg [21], and cardiac output of 4.7 L/min (cardiac input, 2.5 L/min). Cardiac silhouette (*middle picture*) at this time revealed no cardiomegaly. Patient was found to have constrictive pericarditis at surgery, and following pericardectomy he improved dramatically.

usually those with pyelonephritis, obstructive renal disease, and polycystic renal disease, exhibit mild, if any, hypertension because of larger urine outputs and a salt-losing tendency. Normal blood pressure in previously hypertensive patients with other causes of renal failure is in our experience usually secondary to volume depletion. This commonly occurs in patients who are treated with low-salt diets in the face of a fixed renal sodium loss. Also accompanying this "normal" blood pressure may be deterioration in renal function which occasionally can be reversed with the reinstitution of appropriate amounts of sodium in the diet.

The pathophysiology of an elevated blood pressure in patients with end-stage renal disease is different from that of patients with early parenchymal renal disease. A number of studies [113-115] have indicated that in early renal disease, hypertension is associated with an increase in peripheral vascular resistance with minimal, if any, increase in extracellular volume. As renal insufficiency progresses, the role of extracellular volume becomes more important [38,116,117]. A correlation between systolic blood pressure and extracellular volume or total body exchangeable sodium has been found in patients with chronic renal failure [38,118], and this relationship is even more predictable in the anephric patient [59,119-121]. That extracellular volume is important in producing hypertension has become obvious in light of the large number of hypertensive patients whose blood pressure is controllable simply with ultrafiltration while on hemodialysis. Approximately 70 to 75 percent of all hypertensive individuals who have been treated by hemodialysis in our program have become normotensive with hemodialysis and volume reduction. Similar results have been found by others [121-125]. Hampers et al [37] demonstrated that hypertension remained when the patient's weight and intravascular volume were maintained constant, suggesting that reduction in blood pressure with hemodialysis is due to fluid removal and not the dialysis of some hypertension-producing factor. Although multiple factors may complicate the hypertension of patients with chronic renal failure, excessive fluid volume has been clearly shown to be the major one and is promptly relieved by adequate ultrafiltration.

Most patients with chronic renal failure remain asymptomatic with regard to hypertension, although chest roentgenograms may reveal mild enlargement of the cardiac silhouette and electrocardiograms may show changes of left ventricular hypertrophy. With prolonged excessive elevation of blood pressure, symptoms of congestive heart failure, retinopathy, and encephalopathy become prominent. Usually other symptoms of the uremic syndrome appear concomitantly. Occasionally we have instituted hemodialysis in patients with severe hypertension (without prominent symptoms of florid uremia) in order to effect ultrafiltration.

Most patients on our program are allowed an average of 4 to 8 gm of salt per day with fluid intakes of 800 to 1500 ml plus the estimated daily urinary output. This is calculated to allow them to gain approximately 1.5 to 2.0 kg in weight between dialyses. This quantity of fluid is removed by most dialyzers with routine dialysis and thus allows the patient more stable dialysis without large fluctuations of volume and blood pressure. This salt and fluid allowance may be modified in the hypertensive patient to aid in lowering extracellular volume.

As stated above, if the patient is brought down to "dry weight," that is, a maximum reduction in extracellular volume, the symptoms and complications of hypertension will be reversed in most patients. It is not unusual to see hypertensive eye-ground change improvement, diminished heart size, and subsequent improvement in the electrocardiogram after a period of careful fluid control. Maximal ultrafiltration when necessary can be effected during dialysis by increasing the negative pressure on the dialysate side, increasing the pressure on the blood side, increasing the osmolality of the dialysate, or by using dialyzers with a greater capability for ultrafiltration. Newer coil kidneys, for instance, can remove 3 to 6 kg of fluid within a 5- to 6-hr period [126]. These physical principles have been discussed (see Chap. 1).

By bleeding the patient into the dialyzer without return of equal amounts of saline, plasma or blood, more fluid may be removed immediately. Such a technique, when performed slowly, is not hazardous. Care should be taken, however, in the patient with severe anemia or in elderly patients who manifest symptoms of coronary or vascular disease. We have found, as have others [127], that although large amounts of fluid may be ultrafiltered with twice weekly dialysis, hypertension is more readily and smoothly controlled when treated at least three times per week. Although we speak of "dry weight" in patients on chronic dialysis, it is doubtful that patients truly obtain an ideal extracellular volume. This is most apparent in the patient with no edema or hypertension while treated with hemodialysis who quickly loses several more kilograms of body weight following successful renal transplantation.

The mortality rate from nonazotemic malignant hypertension is high, and even moderately elevated blood pressure has been shown in long-term studies to adversely affect mortality [128,129]. Hypertension in uremic patients should be treated as vigorously as in nonuremic individuals. The initial approach as has been stressed is to reduce fluid excess by ultrafiltration. If this is unsuccessful one should judiciously add antihypertensive medications. In our hands, the drug of choice for patients with malignant hypertension is diazoxide which can be given by rapid intravenous push through the arteriovenous shunt or fistula, usually in a single dose of 300 mg. Diazoxide does not complicate the dialysis procedure with erratic changes in blood pressure and often potentiates the effect of other antihypertensive medications. Parenteral hydralazine or methyldopa given in small frequent does has also been very effective and has given smoother and less complicated control than intravenous drugs such as Arfonad. Once blood pressure is controlled with these parenteral drugs, patients may be placed on oral medication with concomitant slow reduction of parenteral administration. Methyldopa, the drug most frequently used, is given orally in dosages of 250 mg to 2 gm each day. These drugs may produce severe hypotension with minimal volume depletion during dialysis, and it may be necessary to administer the antihypertensive medication only on nondialysis days to avoid its interference with the hemodialysis procedure. Oral antihypertensive drugs may often be tapered and discontinued later in the dialysis program as hypertension comes under control with ultrafiltration alone. Propanolol, alone or with hydralazine, as well as newer drugs such as minoxidil are being evaluated in hypertensive patients on hemodialysis; however, comment as to their effectiveness is premature.

Despite aggressive dialysis with adequate removal of fluid and maximum doses of hypertensive medications, hypertension may persist in a small number of dialysis patients. These patient have been shown to respond to bilateral nephrectomy [67,119,120,129,130], particularly when the hypertension is associated with markedly elevated renin levels [121-123,131]. A marked increase in total peripheral resistance has been documented in these patients with hypertension [2,37,66] and for the most part is felt to be due to increased activity of the renin–angiotensin axis. In support of this we have found, as have others [121-123,131,132], very low or absent renin levels following bilateral nephrectomy and resolution of hypertension.

Many of these severely hypertensive patients manifest clinical evidence of malignant hypertension, i.e., grade IV hypertensive retinopathy, encephalopathy, advanced left ventricular hypertrophy with congestive heart failure, and in some cases an aortic insufficiency murmur secondary to cardiac dilatation. Despite receiving aggressive dialysis, these patients do poorly. They exhibit general weakness, obtundation, impaired vision, and refractory congestive heart failure.

Dialysis is often inadequate because of poor blood flows related to unstable blood pressure, which may be the result of the massive doses of antihypertensive medication necessary to control blood pressure between hemodialyses. This picture is often so typical that elevated renin levels can often be predicted beforehand. Patients respond promptly to bilateral nephrectomy with immediate resolution of elevated blood pressure accompanied by dramatic improvement in congestive heart failure and reduction in heart size (Fig. 6). Hypertensive eye grounds also resolve and visual acuity improves promptly. Patients becomes more alert and active, therefore facilitating rehabilitation. In a small number of these patients, an immediate blood pressure response to nephrectomy lasts only a few months before the blood pressure slowly rises again to mildly hypertensive levels. Despite recurrent hypertension, however, patients do not experience the same severe side effects manifested when the diseased kidneys were in place. The dramatic improvement in the clinical picture has led us to perform bilateral nephrectomy early in patients with malignant hypertension, particularly in those patients who develop decreased visual acuity with retinopathy or who require such large doses of antihypertensive medication to control blood pressure that rehabilitation is compromised [133]. Early operation in our hands has been attended by low morbidity and no mortality. The beneficial response to bilateral nephrectomy in such patients far outweighs the disadvantages of loss of kidney tissue—i.e., decreased erythropoiesis and the loss of urine output. It should be pointed out that these patients usually have renal failure of gradual onset (at least 6 months) and do not represent those with immediate renal failure due to malignant hypertension. In cases in which the reversibility of the renal disease is unclear, a more prolonged period of dialysis should be performed before instituting bilateral nephrectomy.

We have observed, as have others [121], a large fluid requirement in some of these patients immediately after surgery and during the first several hemodialyses following bilateral nephrectomy. This is likely due to a relative volume deficit following relief of marked vasoconstriction that accompanies marked hypertension. One must be careful to distinguish this volume deficit, which can be as great as 5 or 6 liters, from acute occult blood loss related to surgery.

The two major types of hypertension in patients with chronic renal insufficiency are therefore related to excessive extracellular volume and to the presence of markedly elevated renin levels. A third small group of individuals may have hypertension with a different etiological mechanism—increased total peripheral resistance may be the primary contributing factor. Conway [134] suggested that there are structural

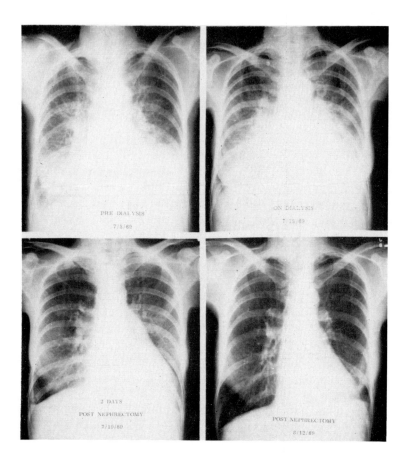

Fig. 6. This 37-year-old patient with malignant hypertension and congestive heart failure unresponsive to diazoxide, diuretics, digoxin, and thoracentesis received 3 hemodialyses with a resultant 10 kg weight loss. Despite dialysis and intensive antihypertensive therapy three was progressive congestive heart failure and persistent malignant hypertension. After bilateral nephrectomy, the patient had prompt amelioration of blood pressure with reduction in heart size, loss of aortic insufficiency murmur, and improvement in cardiovascular symptoms, mentation, and vision.

102

changes encroaching upon the lumen of arterioles throughout the body and this is an important factor in hypertension. The normally reactive vessels (with compromised lumens) would then create greater vascular resistance. The presence of such vascular changes in chronically uremic patients has, however, not been demonstrated. McCubbin et al [135] and Kezdi and Wennemark [136] suggested there may be resetting of baroreceptors in hypertensive patients and this has also been suggested as a cause of hypertension in the uremic, anephric patient [59]. Pickering et al [137] in a study of long-term dialysis patients found decreased reflex sensitivity which changed little at different arterial pressures. They interpreted these data as indicating a resetting of the reflex. In a recent study using the pulse response to pharmacologically induced changes in blood pressure, we were unable to conclusively demonstrate resetting as a cause of hypertension [34]. We found reduced sensitivity of the baroreceptors in both hypertensive and uremic patients and feel this may be important in postural hypotension which many of these patients experienced. The technique, however, was inadequate to support the theory that resetting of the baroreceptor was the *cause* of hypertension.

Increased cardiac output is another potential contributor to hypertension in these patients [3,59,115]. In uremic patients, Neff et al [61] studied the effect of elevated cardiac output and anemia on the development of hypertension. They concluded that increased cardiac output alone was not responsible for the hypertension. We have observed a few young anephric hypertensive patients with clinical signs of hyperdynamism—i.e., bounding pulses and an active precordium—suggesting an increase in cardiac activity. Hypertension in these patients responded dramatically to small doses of propranolol. Propanolol has been reported to be effective in high renin hypertension [138], probably not due to its effect on cardiac output. These patients all had low to absent renin values, and we interpret the control of blood pressure with small doses of propanolol as possible evidence that increased cardiac output was important in the etiology of the hypertension.

Finally, patients may remain hypertensive following nephrectomy because of the presence of a vasoconstrictive substance other than renal renin. While renin is usually low to absent in anephric patients, some investigators have found significant increases in a renin-like enzyme said to be produced from the uterus of anephric females [139]. The importance of small amounts of such a hormone is unknown. Patients with chronic uremia and accelerated hypertension have been shown to have increased aldosterone levels also which correlate with the renin level [140,141]. Aldosterone levels also correlate directly with serum potassium [142,143,144] but have not been found to be significantly elevated in anephric patients; the role of aldosterone in the hypertension of anuric or anephric uremic patients is likewise questionable. Abnormal levels of other hormones implicated in hypertension such as 18-hydroxy-desoxycorticosterone [145] have not been demonstrated in uremic patients. The lack of a substance such as prostaglandin, which is produced by the kidney and is known to have an effect of vasodilatation, is yet to be demonstrated in the uremic or anephric patient. Although there is indeed hypertension in the renoprival state, there is little evidence to support the concept that this "renoprival hypertension" is due directly to absence of renal tissue or some secreted hormone.

Until 1970 it was our policy to perform bilateral nephrectomy in preparation for renal transplantation in all patients. A large number of patients with normal or slightly elevated renin levels, only mildly to moderately elevated blood pressure, and no hypertensive complications underwent bilateral nephrectomy. These patients had a less dramatic response to bilateral nephrectomy than patients with malignant hypertension referred to above [37]. We subsequently reexamined the policy of routine bilateral nephrectomy. A prospective study was initiated in which patients with elevated blood pressure but without significant hypertensive cardiovascular disease, retinopathy, or encephalopathy received transplants without prior bilateral nephrectomy. A recent survey of such post-transplant patients with and without bilateral nephrectomy reveals that hypertension is less common in individuals who previously underwent bilateral nephrectomy. Of 49 patients transplanted without prior nephrectomy, 24 (48 percent) had diastolic pressures greater than 90 mm Hg. The incidence of hypertension in a matched anephric population is 31 percent. Twenty of the 24 hypertensive patients received antihypertensive and/or diuretic medications. Five patients experienced chronic rejection; the remainder had serum creatinine values of less than 2 mg/100 ml. Two patients required bilateral nephrectomy for control of hypertension following transplantation. Hypertension in the remainder was considered controllable with low-dose drug therapy. For this reason *routine* bilateral nephrectomy is no longer performed. At the present time we perform bilateral nephrectomy only in those patients with symptoms and signs of persistent clinical hypertension which interfere with patient rehabilitation or threaten successful transplantation. Bilateral nephrectomy is also performed preoperatively in patients with documented obstructive pyelonephritis with infected urine and patients with polycystic kidney disease who have recurrent bleeding, infection, or a kidney size that interferes mechanically with transplantation.

Other nonhypertensive indications for bilateral nephrectomy include the "emergency" use of bilateral nephrectomy in an attempt to effectively reverse the severe intra-alveolar hemorrhage in patients with Goodpasture's syndrome [146,147]. We have performed bilateral nephrectomy in two such patients with gratifying results. Because hemoptysis in a patient with renal failure is most often due to simple pulmonary edema, the decision to perform nephrectomy should follow an intensive course of hemodialysis and ultrafiltration. Unless death from pulmonary insufficiency is imminent or there is biopsy proof of an intra-alveolar linear deposition consistent with the diagnosis of Goodpasture's syndrome, bilateral nephrectomy should be withheld.

REFERENCES

1. Ueda, H., Sakamoto, T., Sawayama, T.: Clinical and phonocardiographic studies of gallop rhythm. Report II. Re-evaluation of kidney gallop. Jap Heart J 5:201, 1964.
2. Goss, J.E., Alfrey, A.C., Vogel, J.H.K., et al: Hemodynamic changes during hemodialysis. Trans Am Soc Artif Intern Organs 13:68, 1967.
3. Mostert, J.W., Evers, J.L., Hobika, G.A., et al: The haemodynamic response to chronic renal failure as studied in the azotemic state. Br J Anaest 42:397, 1970.
4. Mostert, J.W., Evers, J.L., Hobika, G.H., et al: Cardiac evaluation in renal and pulmonary insufficiency. N Y State J Med 70:1196, 1970.
5. Gibson, D.G.: Haemodynamic factors in the development of acute pulmonary oedema in renal failure. Lancet 2:1217, 1966.
6. Bagdade, J.D., Porte, D., Jr., Bierman, E.L.: Hypertriglyceridemia. A metabolic consequence of chronic renal failure. N Engl J Med 279:181, 1968.
7. Fredrickson, D.S., Levy, R.I., Lees, R.S.: Fat transport in lipoproteins–An integratedapproach to mechanisms and disorders. N Engl J Med 276:273, 1967.
8. Brown, C.E., Richter, I.M.: Medical coronary sclerosis in infancy. Arch Path 31:449, 1941.
9. Katz, A.I., Hampers, C.L., Merrill, J.P.: Secondary hyperparathyroidism and renal osteodystrophy in chronic renal failure. Analysis of 195 patients with observations on the effects of chronic dialysis, kidney transplantation and subtotal parathyroidectomy. Medicine (Baltimore) 48:333, 1969.
10. Moorhead, J.F., Baillod, R.A., Hopewell, J.P., et al: Survival rates of patients treated by home and hospital dialysis and cadaveric renal transplantation. Br Med J 4:83, 1970.
11. Lewin, J., Trautman, L.: Ischemic myocardium damage in chronic renal failure. Br Med J 4:151, 1971.

12. Gore, I., Arons,W.: Calcification of the hyocardium. Arch Path 48:1, 1949.
13. Davidson, R.C., Pendras, J.P.: Calcium-related cardio-respiratory death in chronic hemodialysis. Trans Am Soc Artif Intern Organs 13:36, 1967.
14. Terman, D.S., Alfrey, A.C., Hammond, W.S., et al: Cardiac calcification in uremia. A clinical biochemical and pathologic study. Am J Med 50: 744, 1971.
15. Bailey, G.L., Hampers, C.L., Merrill, J.P.: Reversible cardiomyopathy in uremia. Trans Am Soc Artif Intern Organs 13:263, 1967.
16. Matalon, R., Moussalli, A.R.J., Nodos, B.D., et al: Functional aortic insufficiency—A feature of renal failure. N Engl J Med 285:1522, 1971.
17. Adam, W.R., Dawborn, J.K., Rosenbaum, M.: Transient early diastolic murmurs in patients with renal failure. Med J Aust 2:1085, 1970.
18. Pendras, J.P., Erickson, R.V.: Clinical experience with 16 patients on chronic hemodialysis. Trans Am Soc Artif Intern Organs 11:238, 1965.
19. Hampers, C.L., Schupak, E.: Long-term hemodialysis: The management of the patient with chronic renal failure. New York, Grune & Stratton, 1967, p 65.
20. Goodwin, N.J., Castronuovo, J.J., Friedman, E.A.: Recurrent septic pulmonary embolization complicating maintenance hemodialysis. Ann Intern Med 71:29, 1969.
21. Levi, J., Robson, M., Rosenfeld, J.B.: Septicemia and pulmonary embolism complicating use of arteriovenous fistula in maintenance dialysis. Lancet 2:288, 1970.
22. Smith, C.M., Morton, J.D., Thompson, R.D.: Bacterial endoarteritis. A probably case in an arteriovenous fistula used for long-term hemodialysis. JAMA 210:131, 1969.
23. Brescia, M.J., Cimino, J.E., Appel, K. et al: Chronic hemodialysis using venipuncture and surgically created arteriovenous fistula. N Engl J Med 275:1089, 1966.
24. Goodman, J.S., Crews, H.D., Ginn, H.E., et al: Bacterial endocarditis as a possible complication of chronic hemodialysis. N Engl J Med 280: 876, 1969.
25. King, L.H., Jr., Bradley, K.P., Shires, D.L., Jr., et al: Bacterial endocarditis in chronic hemodialysis patients: A complication more common than previously suspected. Surgery 69:554, 1971.
26. Ribot, S., Gilbert, L., Rothfeld, E.L., et al: Bacterial endocarditis with pulmonary edema necessitating mitral valve replacement in a hemodialysis dependent patient. J Thorac Cardiovasc Surg 62:59, 1971.
27. Saldanha, L.F., Goldman, R., Adashek, K., et al: Treatment of bacterial endocarditis: Complicating hemodialysis. Br Med J 3:92, 1972.
28. Guild, W.R., Bray, M.D., Merrill, J.P.: Hemopericardium with cardiac tamponade in chronic uremia. N Engl J Med 257:230, 1957.
29. Hager, E.B.: Clinical observations of five patients with uremic pericardial tamponade. N Engl J Med 273:304, 1965.
30. Beaudry, C., Nakomoto, S., Kolff, W.J.: Uremic pericarditis and cardiac tamponade in chronic renal failure. Ann Intern Med 64:990, 1966.

31. Traeger, J., Gonin, A., Delahaye, J.P., et al: Pericardite uremique a evolution constrictive subaique. A propos d'une observation anatomo-clinique chez un brightique traite par les epurations extra renales, au long cours. Lyon Med 211:383, 1964.
32. Spaulding, W.B.: Subacute constrictive uremic pericarditis. Arch Intern Med 119:644, 1967.
33. Wolfe, S.A., Bailey, F.G., Collins, J.J.: Constrictive pericarditis following uremic effusion. J Thorac Cardiovasc Surg 63:540, 1972.
34. Lazarus, J.M., Hampers, C.L., Lowrie, E.G., et al: Baroreceptor activity in normotensive and hypertensive uremic patients. Circulation (in press).
35. Bristow, J.D., Honour, A.J., Pickering, G.W., et al: Diminished baroreflex sensitivity in high blood pressure. Circulation 39:48, 1969.
36. Eckberg, D.L., Brabinsky, M., Braunwald, E.: Defective cardiac parasympathetic control in patients with heart disease. N Engl J Med 285: 877, 1971.
37. Hampers, C.L., Skillman, J.J., Lyons, J.H., et al: A hemodynamic evaluation of bilateral nephrectomy and hemodialysis in hypertensive man. Circulation 35:272, 1967.
38. Dustan, H.P., Page, J.A.: Some factors in renal and renoprival hypertension. J Lab Clin Med 64:948, 1964.
39. Schupak, E., Urichek, P., Merrill, J.P.: The long-term maintenance of bilaterally nephrectomized man by periodic hemodialysis. Trans Am Soc Artif Intern Organs 9:24, 1963.
40. Goldenberger, S., Thompson, A., Guha, A.: Autonomic nervous dysfunction in chronic renal failure. Circ Res 19:531, 1971.
41. Lowenthal, D.T., Reidenberg, M.M.: The heart rate response to atropine in uremic patients, obese subjects before and during fasting, and patients with other chronic illnesses. Proc Soc Exp Biol Med 139:390, 1972.
42. Nidus, B.D., Matalon, R., Cantacuzino, D., et al: Uremic pleuritis— A clinicopathological entity. N Engl J Med 281:255, 1969.
43. Binak, K., Regan, T.J., Christensen, R.C., et al: Arteriovenous fistula: Hemodynamic effects of occlusion and exercise. Am Heart J 60:495, 1960.
44. Pate, J.W., Sherman, R.T., Jackson, T., et al: Cardiac failure following traumatic arteriovenous fistula: A report of fourteen cases. J Trauma 5:398, 1965.
45. Holman, E.: Abnormal arteriovenous communications, great variability of effects with particular reference to delayed development of cardiac failure. Circulation 32:1001, 1965.
46. Dotremont, G., Piessens, J., Verberckmoes, et al: Hemodynamic studies in patients on chronic hemodialysis by venipuncture of a peripheral arterio-venous fistula. Acta Cardiol (Brux.) 25:230, 1970.
47. Heidland, A., Klütsch, K., Scheitza, E., et al: Klinische ertahrungen mit der subkutanen arterio-venosen Fistel in der Hämodialyse Behandlung. Dtsch Med Wochenschr 92:427, 1967.
48. Franz, H.E., Roehl, L., Vollmar, J., et al: Chronische Hämodialyse mit Hilfe der Venepunktion und Kunstlich gesetzer AV-Fistel. Verh Dtsch Ges Inn Med 73:997, 1967.

49. Payne, R.M., Soderblom, R.E., Lobstein, P., et al: Exercise-induced hemodynamic effects of arteriovenous fistulas used for hemodialysis. Kidney Internat 2:344, 1972.
50. Klinkman, H., Rohmann, H., Teichmann, G., et al: Influence of an arteriovenous forearm fistula on the circulation of patients with chronic uremia. Proc European Dialysis and Transplant Assoc 4:50, 1967. Excerpta Medica Internat Congress Series #155 (Paris).
51. Lazarthes, F.: Fistules arterio-veineuses chirurgicales et hemodialyse. Imprimarie Fournie (Toulouse), 1969.
52. Menno, A.D., Zizzi, J., Hodson, J., et al: An evaluation of the radial arteriovenous fistula as a substitute for the Quinton shunt in chronic hemodialysis. Trans Am Soc Artif Intern Organs 13:62, 1967.
53. Johnson, G., Blythe, W.D.: Hemodynamic effects of arteriovenous shunts used for hemodialysis. Ann Surg 171:715, 1970.
54. Ackman, C.F.D., Khonsari, H., Mount, B., et al: Arteriovenous fistulae for hemodialysis: Advantage with cadaver renal transplantation. Proc European Dialysis and Transplant Assoc. 4:86, 1967. Excerpta Medica Internat Congress Series #155 (Paris).
55. Hanson, J.S., Carmody, M., Keogh, B., et al: Access to circulation by permanent arteriovenous fistula in regular dialysis treatment. Br Med J 4:586, 1967.
56. Hurwich, B.J.: Plethysmographic forearm blood flow studies in maintenance hemodialysis patients with radial arteriovenous fistulae. Nephron 6:673, 1969.
57. McMillan, R., Evans, D.B.: Experience with three Brescia-Cimino shunts. Br Med J 3:781, 1968.
58. Ahern, D.J., Maher, J.F.: Heart failure as a complication of hemodialysis arteriovenous fistula. Ann Intern Med 77:201, 1972.
59. Merrill, J.P., Schupak, E.: Mechanisms of hypertension in renoprival man. Can Med Assoc J 90:328, 1964.
60. Bower, J.D., Coleman, T.G.: Circulatory function during chronic hemodialysis. Trans Am Soc Artif Intern Organs 15:373, 1969.
61. Neff, M.S., Kim, K.E., Persoff, M., et al: Hemodynamics of uremic anemia. Circulation 43:876, 1971.
62. Kim, K.E., Onesti, G., Schwartz, A.B., et al: Hemodynamic changes in uremia. Abstract #979. Fifth Internat Congress Nephrology, Mexico City, Mexico. 1971.
63. Anthonisen, P., Holst, E.: Determination of cardiac output and other hemodynamic data in uremic patients using dye dilution technique. Scand J Clin Lab Invest 12:481, 1960.
64. Del Greco, F., Shere, J., Simon, N.M.: Hemodynamic effects of hemodialysis in chronic renal failure. Trans Am Soc Artif Intern Organs 10: 353, 1964.
65. Henderson, L.W., Ambrosi, C., Starr, I.: Cardiodynamic studies of uremics before and after dialysis. Nephron 8:511, 1971.
66. Del Greco, F., Simon, N.M., Rogaska, J., et al: Hemodynamic studies in chronic uremia. Circulation 60:87, 1969.

67. Hampers, C.L., Zollinger, R.M., Skillman, J.J., et al: Hemodynamic and body composition changes following bilateral nephrectomy in chronic renal failure. Circulation 40:367, 1969.

68. Kim, K.E., Neff, M., Cohen, B., et al: Blood volume changes and hypotension during hemodialysis. Trans Am Soc Artif Intern Organs 16: 508, 1970.

69. Frohlich, E.D., Bhatia, S., Matter, B.J., et al: Mechanism of acute arterial pressure changes during hemodialysis. J Lab Clin Med 78:1014, 1971.

70. Ackerman, G.L., Doherty, J.E., Flanigan, W.J.: Peritoneal dialysis and hemodialysis of tritiated digoxin. Ann Intern Med 67:718, 1967.

71. Kohn, R.M., Kiley, J.E.: Electrocardiographic changes during hemodialysis, with observations on contribution of electrolyte disturbances to digitalis toxicity. Ann Intern Med 39:38, 1953.

72. Levine, H.D., Wapzer, S.H., Merrill, J.P.: Dialyzable currents of injury in potassium intoxication resembling acute myocardial infarction or pericarditis. Circulation 13:29, 1956.

73. Papadimitriou, M., Roy, R.R., Varkarakis, M.: Electrocardiographic changes and plasma potassium levels in patients on regular hemodialysis. Br Med J 1:268, 1970.

74. Frohnert, P.P., Giuliani, E.R., Freidberg, M., et al: Statistical investigation of correlations between serum potassium levels and electrocardiographic findings in patients on intermittent hemodialysis therapy. Circulation 61:667, 1970.

75. Del Greco, F., Grumer, A.: Electrolyte and electrocardiographic changes in the course of hemodialysis. Am J Cardiol 9:43, 1962.

76. Rubin, A.L., Lubash, G.D., Cohen, B.D., et al: Electrocardiographic changes during hemodialysis with the artificial kidney. Circulation 18:227, 1958.

77. Matalon, R., Nodus, B.D., Eisinger, R.P.: Psuedoarrhythmias during hemodialysis. N Engl J Med 278:1439, 1968.

78. Johnson, W.J., Frohnert, P.P., Novak, P.P.: Potassium balance in patients maintained by long-term hemodialysis against potassium free dialysate. Mayo Clinic & Mayo Foundation; 4th International Congress of Nephrology,(abstract), (Stockholm), 1969, p 303.

79. Seedat, Y.K.: Exchangeable potassium study in patients undergoing chronic hemodialysis. Br Med J 2:344, 1969.

80. Johny, K.U., Lawrence, J.R., Halloran, M.W., et al: Changes in total body potassium and erythrocyte cations during maintenance hemodialysis. Queen Elizabeth Hospital; 4th International Congress of Nephrology, (abstract), (Stockholm), 1969, p 301.

81. Morgan, A.G., Burkinshaw, L., Robinson, P.J.A., et al: Potassium balance and acid-base changes in patients undergoing regular hemodialysis therapy. Br Med J 1:779, 1970.

82. Hampers, C.L., Bailey, G.L., Hager, E.B., et al: Major surgery in patients on maintenance hemodialysis. Am J Surg 115:747, 1968.

83. Wacker, W., Merrill, J.P.: Uremic pericarditis in acute and chronic renal failure. JAMA 156:764, 1954.
84. Skov, P.E., Hansen, H.E., Spencer, E.S.: Uremic pericarditis. Acta Med Scand 186:421, 1965.
85. Bailey, G.L., Hampers, C.L., Hager, E.B., et al: Uremic pericarditis: Clinical features and management. Circulation 38:582, 1968.
86. Barach, A.L.: Pericarditis in chronic nephritis. Am J Med Sci 163:44, 1972.
87. Richter, A.B., O'Hare, J.P.: Heart in chronic glomerulonephritis. N Engl J Med 214:824, 1936.
88. Bright, R.: Tabular view of the morbid appearances in 100 cases connected with albuminous urine; with observations. Guys Hosp Rep 1:338, 1936.
89. Richter, A.B.: Pericarditis in uremia. J Indiana State Med Assoc 29:369, 1936.
90. Comty, C.M., Cohen, S.L., Shapiro, F.L.: Pericarditis in chronic uremia and its sequels. Ann Intern Med 75:173, 1971.
91. Gouley, B.A.: Myocardial degeneration associated with uremia in advanced hypertensive disease and chronic glomerular nephritis. Am J Med Sci 200:39, 1940.
92. Langendorf, R., Pirani, C.L.: Heart in uremia: electrocardiographic and pathologic study. Am Heart J 33:282, 1949.
93. Hampers, C.L., Blaufox, M.D., Merrill, J.P.: Anticoagulation rebound after hemodialysis. N Engl J Med 275:776, 1966.
94. Keith, N.M., Pruitt, R.D., Baggenstoss, A.H.: Electrocardiographic changes in pericarditis associated with uremia. Am Heart J 31:527, 1946.
95. Goodman, C.J., Brown, H.: Report of two cases of cardiac tamponade in uremic pericarditis. JAMA 162:1459, 1956.
96. Buja, M., Friedman, C.A., Roberts, W.C.: Hemorrhagic pericarditis in uremia. Arch Path 90:325, 1970.
97. Alfrey, A.C., Gloss, J.E., Ogden, D.A., et al: Uremic hemopericardium. Am J Med 45:391, 1968.
98. Collins, H.A., Killen, D.A., Gobbel, W.G., et al: Pericardectomy for uremic pericardial tamponade. Ann Thorac Surg 9:327, 1970.
99. Stone, J.R., Martin, R.A.: Bloody pericardial fluid or intracardiac blood. A method for quick and accurate differentiation. Ann Intern Med 77:592, 1972.
100. Moss, A.J., Bruhn, F.: The echocardiogram. An ultrasound technique for the detection of pericardial effusion. N Engl J Med 274:380, 1966.
101. Pridie, R.B., Turnbull, T.A.: Diagnosis of pericardial effusion by ultrasound. Br Med J 3:356, 1968.
102. Feigenbaum, H., Zaky, A., Waldhousen, J.A.: Use of reflected ultrasound in detecting pericardial effusion. Am J Cardiol 19:84, 1967.
103. Paul, R.E., Durant, T.M., Oppenheimer, M.J., et al: Intravenous carbon dioxide for intracardiac gas contrast in the roentgen diagnosis of pericardial effusion and thickening. Am J Roentgenol 78:224, 1957.

104. Scatliff, J.H., Kummer, A.J., Janzen, A.H.: Diagnosis of pericardial effusion with intracardiac carbon dioxide. Radiology 73:871, 1959.
105. Williams, R.G., Steinberg, I.: The value of angiocardiography in establishing the diagnosis of pericarditis with effusion. Am J Roentgenol Radium Ther Nucl Med 61:41, 1949.
106. Pyle, R.: Diagnosis of pericardial effusion by intravenous arteriography. N Engl J Med 275:816, 1966.
107. Cohen, M.B., Gral, T., Sokol, A., et al: Pericardial effusion in chronic uremia—Detection by photoscanning. Arch Intern Med 122:404, 1968.
108. Rexman, T.A.: Subacute constrictive uremic pericarditis. Am J Med 46:972, 1969.
109. Lindsay, J., Jr., Crawley, I.S., Callaway, G.M.: Chronic constrictive pericarditis following uremic hemopericardium. Am Heart J 79:390, 1970.
110. Cutforth, R., Freeman, J., Mitchell, R.M.: Uremic constrictive pericarditis. Med J Aust 2:239, 1969.
111. Moraski, R.E., Bousuaros, G.: Constrictive pericarditis due to chronic uremia. N Engl J Med 281:542, 1969.
112. Nickey, W.A., Chinitz, J.L., Flynn, J.J., et al: Surgical correction of uremic constrictive pericarditis. Ann Intern Med 75:222, 1971.
113. Glazer, G.A.: Haemodynamic changes in symptomatic renal hypertension. Cor Vasa 6:264, 1964.
114. DeFazio, V., Christensen, R.C., Regan, T.J., et al: Circulatory changes in acute glomerulonephritis. Circulation 20:190, 1959.
115. Frohlich, E.D., Tarazi, R.C., Dustan, H.P.: Re-examination of the hemodynamics of hypertension Am J Med Sci 257:9, 1969.
116. Merrill, J.P., Giordano, C., Heetderks, D.R.: The role of the kidney in human hypertension. I. Failure of hypertension to develop in the renoprival subject. Am J Med 31:931, 1961.
117. Blumberg, A., Nelp, W.B., Hegstrom, R.M., et al: Extracellular volume in patients with chronic renal disease treated for hypertension by sodium restriction. Lancet 2:69, 1967.
118. Friis, T., Nielsen, B., Willumsen, J.: Total exchangeable sodium in chronic nephropathy with and without hypertension. Acta Med Scand 188:65, 1970.
119. Kolff, W.J., Nakamoto, S., Poutasse, E.F., et al: Effect of bilateral nephrectomy and kidney transplantation on hypertension in man. Circulation II(suppl 2):23, 1964.
120. Onesti, G., Swartz, C., Ramirez, O., et al: Bilateral nephrectomy for control of hypertension in uremia. Trans Am Soc Artif Intern Organs 14:361, 1968.
121. Wilkinson, R., Scott, D.F., Uldall, P.R., et al: Plasma renin and exchangeable sodium in the hypertension of chronic renal failure. Q J Med 34:377, 1970.
122. Vertes, V., Cangiano, J.L., Berman, L.B., et al: Hypertension in end-stage renal disease. N Engl J Med 280:978, 1969.

123. Weidmann, P., Maxwell, M.A., Lupu, A.N., et al: Plasma renin activity and blood pressure in terminal renal failure. N Engl J Med 285:757, 1971.

124. Hegstrom, R.M., Murray, J.S., Pendras, J.P., et al: Two years' experience with periodic hemodialysis in treatment of chronic uremia. Trans Am Soc Artif Intern Organs 8:266, 1962.

125. Comty, C., Rottka, H., Shaldon, S.: Blood pressure control in patients with end-stage renal failure treated by intermittent hemodialysis. Proc Europ Dialysis and Transplant Assoc 1:209, 1964.

126. Lazarus, J.M., Neff, M.S., Schupak, E., et al: The ultra flow II dialyzer. 18th Annual Meeting(abstract), Am Soc Artif Intern Organs, 1972, p 29.

127. Papadimitrious, M., Chisholm, G.D., Shackman, R.: Hypertension in patients on regular hemodialysis and after renal allotransplantation. Lancet 1:902, 1969.

128. Breckenridge, A., Dollery, C.T., Parry, E.H.O.: Prognosis of treated hypertension. Changes in life expectancy and causes of death between 1952 and 1967. Q J Med 39:411, 1970.

129. Veteran's Administration Cooperative Study Group on Antihypertensive Agents: Effects of treatment on morbidity in hypertension. II. Results in patients with diastolic blood pressure averaging 90-114 mm Hg. JAMA 213:1143, 1970.

130. Seto, D., Fritz, W., Nakamoto, S., et al: The effect of bilateral nephrectomy and of sodium and water content on hypertension. Trans Am Soc Artif Intern Organs 9:35, 1963.

131. Toussaint, C., Verniory, A., Cremer, M., et al: Blood renin level in terminal Bright's disease treated by hemodialysis and by renal allotransplantation. International Congress Series #179, Europ Dialysis and Transpl Assoc Proc. 5th Conference, 1968 (Amsterdam); Excerpta Medica, 1969, p 186.

132. Berman, L.B., Vertes, V., Miltra, S., et al: Renin-angiotensin system inanephric patients. N Engl J Med 286:58-61, 1972.

133. Lazarus, J.M., Hampers, C.L., Bennett, A.H., et al: Urgent bilateral nephrectomy for severe hypertension. Ann Intern Med 76:733, 1972.

134. Conway, J.: Vascular reactivity in experimental hypertension measured after hexamethonium. Circulation 17:807, 1958.

135. McCubbin, J.W., Green, J.H., Page, I.H.: Baroreceptor function in chronic renal hypertension. Circ Res 4:205, 1956.

136. Kezdi, P., Wennermark, J.R.: Baroreceptor and synthetic activity in experimental renal hypertension in the dog. Circulation 17:785, 1958.

137. Pickering, T.G., Gribbin, B., Oliver, D.O.: Baroreflex sensitivity in patients on long-term hemodialysis. Clin Sci 42:10P, 1972.

138. Buhler, F.R., Laragh, J.H., Baer, L., et al: Propranolol inhibition of renin secretion. A specific approach to diagnosis and treatment of renin-dependent hypertensive diseases. N Engl J Med 287:1209, 1972.

139. Capelli, J.P., Wesson, L.G., Aponte, G.E., et al: Characterization and source of a renin-like enzyme in anephric humans. J Clin Endocrinol Metab 28:221, 1968.

140. Weidmann, P., Maxwell, M.H., Lupu, A.N.: Plasma aldosterone in terminal renal failure. Ann Intern Med 78:13, 1973.
141. Laragh, J.H., Ulik, S., Januszewicz, V., et al: Aldosterone secretion and primary and malignant hypertension. J Clin Invest 39:1092, 1960.
142. Mitra, S., Genuth, S.M., Berman, L.B., et al: Aldosterone secretion in anephric patients. N Engl J Med 286:61, 1972.
143. Williams, G.H., Bailey, G.L., Hampers, C.L., et al: Studies on the metabolism of aldosterone in chronic renal failure and in anephric man. Kidney Int (in press).
144. Bayard, F., Cooke, C.R., Tiller, D.J., et al: The regulation of aldosterone secretion in anephric man. J Clin Invest 50:1585, 1971.
145. Melby, J.C., Dale, S.L., Wilson, T.E.: 18-hydroxy-deoxycorticosterone in human hypertension. Circ Res 28 & 29 (suppl 2):143, 1971.
146. Maddock, R.K., Jr.., Stevens, L.E., Reemtsma, K., et al: Goodpasture's syndrome: Cessation of pulmonary hemmorhage after bilateral nephrectomy. Ann Intern Med 67:1258, 1967.
147. Nowakowski, A., Grove, R.B., King, L.H., Jr., et al: Goodpasture's syndrome: Recovery from severe pulmonary hemorrhage after bilateral nephrectomy. Ann Intern Med 75:243, 1971.

6

The Hematopoietic System

THE RED CELL

Anemia is inevitably present in patients with severe chronic renal failure and in some may cause troublesome symptoms. Many patients tolerate marked degrees of anemia well and only rarely require transfusions. Others, however, require frequent blood administration even if transfusions are given only for symptomatic anemia. Transfusion therapy may be attended by complications such as transfusion reactions and sensitization to certain leukocyte-transplantation antigens. Hepatitis may also be a formidable complication in a hemodialysis unit. Therefore, therapy must be individualized and blood administration avoided whenever possible.

Currently, bone marrow failure is believed to be the primary physiologic abnormality in the anemia of renal failure. A mild degree of premature red cell destruction further complicates a relatively hypoplastic erythron. There is a loose correlation between the degree of anemia and the severity of renal disease as measured by the BUN, serum creatinine, and creatinine clearance [1,2]. Generally, only mild anemia may appear as creatinine clearance falls toward 25 ml/min, but when clearance falls below this value anemia tends to become much more severe. The correlations, however, are loose and much individual variation is observed.

Red cell morphology is usually normocytic and normochromic, and bone marrow examination may reveal a slightly hypercellular marrow with "normal" erythropoiesis. For the degree of anemia usually present one would expect increased erythroid activity, but hypercellularity, if present, mainly involves the myeloid and megakaryocytic cells [3]. In some instances erythroid hypoplasia or delayed maturation is also observed.

"Burr" cells have been noted in the peripheral blood [4] and may be a common finding [5]. In addition, macrocytosis may occur in from 10 to 15 percent of cases [3]. Hypersegmented polymorphonuclear leukocytes may also be seen [6]. The salts of folic acid are water soluble, of relatively low molecular weight (mol wt, 441), and are only about two-thirds bound to plasma proteins. As such, folate in the serum would be expected to be dialyzable, and indeed this has been demonstrated to be so [6,7]. Serum folate levels in individuals undergoing chronic hemodialysis may be low if dietary intake is inadequate. Erythrocyte folic acid levels, on the other hand, are usually normal even if accompanying plasma levels are low [7]. A slow release of folic acid from stores has been postulated as the explanation for this phenomenon and may be a factor that offsets folic acid loss during dialysis. There is unfortunately no clear or well-defined explanation for this slow release. Conversely, vitamin B-12 is a larger molecule (mol wt, 1355) and is more highly protein bound. It is therefore minimally dialyzable [6,7] and serum levels are usually within normal limits.

A serum factor capable of stimulating erythropoiesis in recipient animals was first demonstrated in 1953 [8]. Subsequently, Jacobson and colleagues [9] suggested that the kidney was the site of production of this erythropoietic-stimulating factor (ESF). Neats [10] found that bilateral nephrectomy markedly diminished the number of erythroblasts in the marrow and caused a reduction in iron turnover. But bilateral ureteral ligation resulting in the same level of azotemia, failed to reduce erythroblasts in the marrow. Furthermore, iron turnover, although slightly reduced, was significantly higher than in the nephrectomized group. This suggests that the kidneys are essential in maintaining normal erythropoiesis, and chemical uremia per se is not the sole factor causing the anemia of chronic renal failure.

The kidney is currently considered the main source of production or activation of erythropoietin. Current evidence suggests that a substance termed renal erythropoietic factor (REF) is produced in the kidney and this factor, which does not resemble erythropoietin chemically, is capable of generating active erythropoietin from a substance circulating in the serum [11]. REF appears to be an enzyme that cleaves part of a serum substrate to generate functional erythropoietin. The system is analogous, then, to the renin–angiotensin system.

Animal experiments have shed some light on the role of the kidney in erythropoiesis [12]. A progressive decline in the erythropoietin level of anephric, hypoxic rats results in no detectable activity approximately 18 hours after nephrectomy. Nephrectomized rats are unable to mount an erythropoietin response to hypoxia, while animals made uremic by bilateral ureteral ligation are capable of a normal response. Intravenous injection of REF restores the ability of nephrectomized animals to increase serum erythropoietin in response to hypoxia. This indicates that some substrate synthesized at least partly in extrarenal sites remains in these nephrectomized animals.

Anephric individuals on chronic hemodialysis may be maintained without repeated blood transfusions. This clinical observation and the studies of Nathan and colleagues [13] suggest that a low level of erythropoiesis is possible even in the absence of renal tissue per se. The normoblast percentage in the marrow, used as an index of erythropoietin activity, falls markedly from 5 to 100 days after bilateral nephrectomy, but a low level of erythropoiesis is maintained [14]. Further supporting the concept of an extrarenal erythropoietic-stimulating factor(s) is the rare demonstration of ESF in the serum of anephric individuals [15,16].

Most anemic patients with normal renal function exhibit elevations of plasma erythropoietin. It is uncommon, however, for a measurable titer of ESF to be found in equally anemic but uremic patients [17,18]. Nevertheless, detectable levels are occasionally found [13,17,18]. While ESF activity is low for the degree of anemia commonly encountered, as noted earlier, the marrow of animals made uremic by nephrectomy seems capable of responding to parenteral ESF [19]. No existing evidence suggests that dialysis enhances the ability of a uremic individual to manufacture ESF [20]. However, renal transplantation, despite denervation of the kidney, restores the ESF response to anemia [21]. There is no absolute correlation between the usual parameters of renal function and the ability of the allograft to elaborate erythropoietin [21].

Iron turnover studies have been used extensively to investigate the anemia of renal failure [16,20,22-28]. While there appears to be no defect in the gastrointestinal absorption of iron [22], marrow iron utilization is severely impaired. In general, total plasma-iron turnover (PIT)—expressed in milligrams per 100 milliliters of whole blood per day—is considered to be composed of erythroid-iron turnover (EIT) and a nonerythroid component [23]. EIT represents the amount of iron utilized in the manufacture of red blood cells per day. The red cell utilization (RCU) of iron represents the fraction of a dose of radioiron ultimately used in the manufacture of red blood cells. Normal values for PIT, RCU, and EIT in nonanemic individuals are approximately 0.70 mg/100 ml whole blood per day, 80 percent, and 0.56 mg/100 ml whole blood per day, respectively [23]. Patients with hemolytic anemia and hematocrit levels in the range of those commonly associated with chronic renal failure may be expected to show plasma and erythroid iron turnovers in excess of 2.0 and 1.5 mg/100 ml whole blood per day, respectively. Presumably marrow function is near normal in these individuals. Patients with chronic renal failure, on the other hand, rarely exhibit such elevated values. Iron turnover has uniformly been shown to be low in these patients [16,23-28]. When hematocrit levels average between 19 and 30 vol%, it is not uncommon to observe PIT rates in the range of 0.8 mg/100 ml whole blood per day [12,23,24,28]. While iron turnover in uremic patients with anemia falls within the normal range for individuals with normal red cell volumes, it is inordinately low considering the degree of anemia usually present. The anemia of renal failure may therefore be classified as hypoproliferative.

Patients with renal failure seem to fall into two broad categories that correlate with findings of iron overload [23,24]. The first group is characterized by relatively normal plasma-iron concentrations and normal transferrin saturations. Marrow iron tends to be normal in amount, and EIT—while low considering the degree of anemia—is relatively normal for individuals who have normal red cell volumes. RCU is normal (80 percent) and transfusion requirements are minimal. The second group typically exhibits findings of iron overload with high serum-iron concentrations and high transferrin saturation. RCU and EIT are inordinately low (approximately 35 percent and 0.3 mg/100 ml whole blood per day, respectively). Transfusion requirements in this group tend to be quite high. Unfortunately, there is no clear explanation for this difference and no current hypothesis to suggest why some patients fall into one group and some into the other.

While erythropoiesis is at a low level with kidneys in situ, removal of the diseased organs further compromises the patient's ability to manufacture red blood cells. Van Ypersele de Strihou and Stragier [29] have shown that transfusion requirements increase and average hematocrit levels decrease after removal of the kidneys in chronic hemodialysis patients. A similar observation has been described by Kominami and colleagues [16]. Figure 1 illustrates these findings. EIT uniformly falls after nephrectomy even though the severity of renal failure prior to surgery is sufficient to require hemodialysis. Figure 2 illustrates this observation and shows that the magnitude of the fall

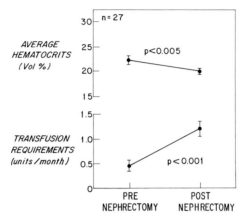

Fig. 1. Average hematocrit levels and mean transfusion requirements in 27 patients before and after bilateral nephrectomy. Divisions indicate S.E.M.

is proportional to the prenephrectomy value. This phenomenon would be expected if kidney removal effected a reduction in erythropoietic activity to some basal value. The conclusion that removal of diseased kidneys adversely affects hematopoiesis is inescapable. Nephrectomy should be reserved for specific indications (e.g., severe hypertension or symptomatic infection) which were covered more fully in Chapter 5.

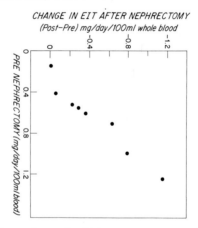

Fig. 2. Change in erythroid-iron turnover rate after nephrectomy (postnephrectomy value minus prenephrectomy value) is correlated with prenephrectomy turnover rate. This observation suggests that EIT falls to some basal level after kidneys are removed.

From the foregoing, it seems reasonable to assume that hypo-proliferative anemia characteristic of chronic renal failure may be due mainly to a lack of erythropoietic activity in the blood. Nonetheless, some studies have suggested that uremic serum may contain an inhibitor of marrow activity. Suspension cultures of marrow from normal individuals have been incubated in sera from patients with anemia and renal failure. The proportion of hemoglobinized normoblasts in these cultures is significantly less than in control cultures after 24 hours [30]. Berman and Powsner [31] also found that azotemic plasma inhibited the maturation of marrow cells from normal individuals. In addition, they found that marrow cells from individuals with azotemia matured more rapidly when incubated in a medium containing normal rather than azotemic plasma. The studies suggest that plasma factors may partially inhibit normoblast maturation in chronic renal failure.

Thorup and colleagues [32] and Erslev and Hughes [33] have pre-sented data suggesting that the rate of iron removal from a culture medium by suspension of cells procured from patients with chronic renal failure is below expected values. Uremic serum, furthermore, inhibits iron uptake in cultures of normal marrow cells. In these studies, the uptake of iron was estimated by counting an aliquot of cells and dividing by the counted number of cells in the aliquot, rather than by counting radioactivity in individual cells. In contrast, Markson and Moore [34] used autoradiographic techniques and presented data sug-gesting that the uptake of radioactive iron, glycine, formate, and methionine by individual normoblasts is normal. Marrow from normal individuals was incubated with sera from uremic patients. Uptake of all the above-mentioned isotopes was comparable to the uptake of control cultures. In addition, marrow from uremic patients was incu-bated in culture with uremic sera and the uptake of ^{59}Fe by normoblasts was also normal. The authors concluded that the synthesis of neither hemoglobin nor DNA by individual normoblasts is inhibited by uremic sera in suspension cultures. This observation is in marked contrast to in vivo ferrokinetic studies. The apparent paradox could most easily be explained on the basis of marrow cellularity. In the uremic patient, poor utilization of iron might be caused by a relatively hypocellular, immature marrow, whereas in culture the uptake per cell would be normal. As previously noted marrow cellularity is usually normal although low for the prevailing anemia. Individual normoblast's iron uptake in culture does not necessarily indicate normal hemoglobin synthesis—it is possible that the initial incorporation of iron into the cell is normal but the final synthesis of hemoglobin could be inhibited somehow. This explanation is consistent with the observed inhibition of normoblast maturation by uremic serum [30,31].

Suppression of activity in these cell culture systems must be interpreted cautiously. Uremic serum has been shown to be toxic for HeLa cells in tissue culture [35]. Uremic serum, furthermore, has been shown both to suppress [36] and have no effect on [37] cultures of fibroblasts. Therefore, any effects on marrow culture may be nonspecific. There may be a toxic suppression of the marrow or a coexisting deficiency of some other substance in uremia as well as a deficiency in ESF. The data on this point are not completely clear and further work is required.

Hemodialysis may provide some benefit to hematopoiesis in the uremic individual. It is clear, however, that hemodialysis rarely causes hematocrit levels to rise to normal values, except in patients with polycystic renal disease. Mann and colleagues [20], who have studied iron turnover rates in patients before and after peritoneal dialysis, collected data suggesting that PIT may indeed increase after dialysis. However, iron deficiency appears to have been corrected concomitantly in most of their patients, and this—rather than dialysis in and of itself—may have been the cause for improvement. The data of Kurtides and colleagues [38] suggest that iron turnover may improve after a single dialysis, but the values presented do not approach those expected for normal individuals with a similar degree of anemia. Eshbach and co-workers [28] studied 16 patients with advanced renal disease under dialysis therapy for as long as 6 years. Five of these patients were restudied from 1 to 3 years after the initial study. In general, EIT increased from an average of 0.36 to 0.73 mg/100 ml whole blood per day. In essence, this constitutes a doubling of erythropoietic function, although even the improved level is below that expected for the degree of anemia. In 4 of the 5 patients, iron overload receded with increasing EIT and red blood cell production. While hematocrit level improved, it remained far below the normal value.

Testosterone therapy has been suggested as a useful agent to increase hematocrit levels and improve ferrokinetics, thereby reducing transfusion requirements [39,40]. The response in individual patients, however, may be inconsistent and excellent results may be obtained in some individuals while relatively little effect is produced in others. Furthermore, such therapeutic complications such as priapism in men, hirsutism in women, and hepatic dysfunction in both sexes may occur. Favorable response to androgen therapy has been reported in anephric patients as well as in individuals with kidneys in situ [39,41,42]. Animal studies support the observation that erythropoietin secreted from extrarenal sites may be stimulated by androgens [43]. Male rats exhibit a significantly greater erythropoietin response to an hypoxic stimulus than do female rats. A similar difference is noted in nephrectomized animals. The difference in both renal and extrarenal erythropoietin production of male and female animals was abolished by castration of the male. Castration of the female resulted in a rise in erythropoietin levels of rats with intact kidneys, but not in anephric rats. These results have been interpreted as suggesting that extrarenal sites of erythropoietin are sensitive to the action of androgens, but to a lesser extent than are renal sites. Of general and possibly therapeutic interest is the observation that the erythropoietic effects of testosterone in rats may be completely abolished by phenobarbital pretreatment [44]. Barbiturates may then significantly blunt the erythropoietic effects of testosterone in patients undergoing chronic hemodialysis.

Iron therapy has been suggested for patients maintained on chronic hemodialysis. The usual blood loss which attends hemodialytic therapy may be highly variable [45]. Furthermore, blood sampling constitutes another source of iron loss. Normal dietary intake may be insufficient to compensate for this loss, and some centers recommend the routine administration of small doses of oral iron [46].

Emerson [47], in 1948, was the first to demonstrate reduced red blood cell survival in patients with anemia associated with glomerulonephritis. He recognized that the degree of hemolysis should have been compensated for by a normally responsive marrow and that reduced red blood cell production must have been a major factor in the genesis of the patient's anemia. Since that time, numerous studies have documented the hemolysis which may accompany azotemia [25-28,38,48]. Reduced red blood cell survival is not a universal finding, however. Joske et al [26], for example, documented red blood cell destruction in only 4 of 15 cases, and Ragen and colleagues [48] found normal radiochromium half-lives in 14 of 16 patients with chronic renal disease. DesForges and Dawson [25] found that a moderate degree of hemolysis was very common. Conversely, studies on patients undergoing chronic hemodialysis [16,28,38] demonstrate nearly universal reduction in red cell survival. While this reduction is moderate, most investigators feel that it cannot be solely explained by the blood loss which accompanies routine hemodialysis.

Slight abnormalities in mechanical and osmotic fragility may be observed in some patients, but these tests are generally within normal limits [25,27]. Red blood cells taken from uremic individuals who exhibit an in vivo short red blood cell survival exhibit normal survival when transfused into a normal individual [26,27]. Such studies suggest that a defect in red blood cell survival which attends uremia is not intrinsic to the cells themselves but is due to some extra-erythrocytic factor.

Giovannetti and colleagues have demonstrated increased auto-hemolysis and erythrocyte potassium loss in blood from uremic subjects [49]. The autohemolysis was significantly reduced when uremic erythrocytes were incubated in compatible, fresh, normal serum or when uremic blood was first dialyzed in vitro. Erythrocytes from normal subjects showed increased autohemolysis when incubated in sera from uremic patients. The findings suggest that spontaneous in vitro autohemolysis in uremic patients is due to an extracorpuscular factor which may be at least partially removed by dialysis. Welt and colleagues [50,51] have shown that there is a population of uremic subjects with relatively high intraerythrocytic concentrations of sodium. These patients seem to have diminished "pump activity" with a resulting inability to remove sodium from the cell. The net result would then be potassium efflux similar to that described by Giovannetti [49]. The plasma of this group of uremic patients contains a substance which can induce a defect in the ouabain-sensitive ATPase of normal ery-throcytes. Ouabain-sensitive ATPase has been shown to be closely related to the active transport of sodium and potassium that take place at the cell membrane. The metabolic defect seems to be reversible by hemodialysis [52] or by treatment of the uremia [51].

In spite of the observation that there may be a dialyzable factor in the plasma of some uremic patients that enhances autohemolysis, clinical hemodialysis does not seem to improve red blood cell survival [28,38]. Also, bilateral nephrectomy has neither an aggravating nor a salutory effect on the rate of red blood cell destruction [16].

Hyde and Sadler [53] have studied dialysis-induced hemolysis by recirculating blood through several types of hemodialyzers. These included standard parallel plate and twin-coil devices. In vitro evalua-tion showed that the models tested produced only slight hemolysis. Mean plasma-free hemoglobin rose only slightly above control (blood pump alone) values. Nonetheless, these studies were performed by measuring serum hemoglobin concentration and such measurements do not rule out a sublethal erythrocyte injury. Indeglia and colleagues [43] have demonstrated that blood which has been exposed to trauma such as pressure, occlusion, shear or wall interaction exhibits a signifi-cantly shorter red blood cell survival when retransfused into the same animal than blood which has not been so traumatized. This occurs despite minimal immediate hemolysis and the reduced survivals were not proportional to the plasma-hemoglobin increment observed during trauma. Subsequent studies [55] have suggested that the release of several lipid and phospholipid components of erythrocyte membranes accompany mechanical trauma. Trauma may therefore induce varying degrees of cell wall injury which subsequently leads to in vivo destruction of the cell. Bernstein [56] has further shown that erythrocytes from normal and from glucose-6 phosphate-dehydroginase deficient individuals show significant increases in the rate of red cell glucose utilization, CO_2 production, and aerobic metabolism after surface-induced trauma despite immediate hemolysis of only a very small fraction of cells. Increased glucose utilization and Heinz-body production indicated intracellular oxidative damage. This damage appears to be surface and shear mediated and occurs in laminar flow systems. Turbulent flow is not required to produce cell injury [57].

Recently an inhibitor of red cell hexose-monophosphate shunt metabolism has been described in some but not all uremic patients [58]. This appears to be a macromolecular substance slowly dialyzable in vitro that sensitizes the patient to oxidant drugs such as primaquine, sulfonamides, and antimalarials. Ascorbate test G6PD screening is abnormal. The investigators observed that the metabolic defect regularly worsened with hemodialysis against dialysate made with tap water. If deionized water was used, the defect was markedly improved. Patients who exhibited this defect also had foreshortened red blood cell survival. Further clarification of these observations will be of great interest.

Rarer complications of hemodialysis that induce hemolysis have also been reported and are of general interest. If copper tubing is a component of dialysate-making equipment, exhaustion of deionizers may allow acid water to be delivered to this tubing resulting in an increased dialysate copper level. Copper intoxication has been reported and acute hemolysis may be included in the clinical picture [59]. In addition, toxic methemoglobinemia has been reported in a home dialysis patient after nitrate contamination of well water used to make dialysate [60].

Recently splenectomy has been suggested as a possible therapeutic tool for dialysis patients who because they are severely anemic require an inordinate number of transfusions [61,62]. Candidates generally have had enlarged spleens, persistent anemia, and evidence of the splenic trapping of red blood cells on [51]chromium-tagged red cell sequestration studies. Splenectomy reportedly reduces transfusion requirements and increases average hematocrit concentrations in these patients [61,62]. Of the 9 patients in these 2 reports who had both pre- and post-splenectomy red blood cell survival studies, one improved to normal values, 5 improved but still had short survival, and 2 experienced no significant improvement in this parameter. Blendis and colleagues [63] have studied patients with hemodilutional anemia and splenomegaly. Some patients had mild to moderate anemia but normal red blood cell masses indicating that plasma volume was increased. Splenectomy effected a slight fall or no change in the red cell mass, a marked fall in plasma volume, and a rise in hematocrit level. More work is required to discern whether the favorable results of splenectomy in some patients are due to removal of a large spleen which may induce some hemodilutional effects [63] or due to reduced destruction of cells.

Many patients with chronic renal failure tolerate very low hematocrit levels quite well. Certain mechanisms which are compensatory in anemia and serve to increase oxygen transport have recently been described [64]. In otherwise normal individuals, 2,3-diphosphoglycerate (DPG) concentrations within red blood cells have been shown to increase with the onset of anemia. DPG is synthesized by anaerobic glycolysis and is able to enter the core of the hemoglobin molecule between the beta chains. It binds to these, but only when hemoglobin is in the deoxy form. Increased intracellular DPG shifts the hemoglobin-oxygen dissociation curve to the right and allows the red cell to give up oxygen more easily. Elevated levels of organic phosphates, including DPG, within azotemic red blood cells have been described [65,66]. Intracellular 2, 3-DPG is correlated with plasma phosphate concentration and can be increased in normal cells by adding phosphate to plasma or by placing normal cells in uremic, hyperphosphatemic plasma [66].

Mitchell and Pegrum [67] studied the position of the oxygen dissociation curve of hemoglobin in normal subjects and anemic patients with chronic renal failure. Most individuals exhibited right-shifted oxygen dissociation curves and there was a correlation between the degree of anemia and the ease with which the patient's hemoglobin released oxygen. Patients with chronic renal failure on hemodialysis, then, seem to be able to compensate for anemia with increased red blood cell oxygen release in a fashion similar to normal individuals. The administration of testosterone tends to increase erythrocyte DPG and as such may facilitate oxygen delivery to the peripheral tissues [68]. Unfortunately, determinations of the shape of the oxygen dissociation curve and the ease with which hemoglobin releases oxygen in uremic patients treated with testosterone was not determined.

In summary the anemia of chronic renal failure is due primarily to a lack of circulating erythropoietic-stimulating factor. In addition, the marrow may be intrinsically somewhat unresponsive to ESF due to some as yet undefined toxic or deficiency state. The combination of these effects leads to a hypoproliferative anemia. Hemolysis plays some role, but is inconsistent and when present is usually only moderate in severity. Hemodialysis may somewhat improve, but does not normalize, erythropoiesis. Several factors such as the loss of blood attending hemodialysis and sublethal erythrocyte injury may serve to increase the rate of red blood cell destruction coincident with the onset of hemodialysis. This is not usually a major clinical problem, however. Successful renal transplantation generally produces a normal erythropoietic response and therefore normal marrow activity.

WHITE BLOOD CELLS

In contrast to the available literature concerning the anemia of chronic renal failure, information regarding leukocyte function in patients with azotemia or patients undergoing hemodialysis is relatively sparse. Generally, the peripheral blood leukocyte and differential counts are within normal limits [3]. The bone marrow is usually normal or exhibits a mild increase in myeloid: erythroid ratio [3,16], probably due to a relative decrease in the erythroid element. Peripheral blood leukocytes may reveal hypersegmentation thought to be due to a relative folate deficiency [6,7,69].

Little is known about polymorphonuclear leukocyte function in azotemic patients. Alexander and colleagues [70] have studied the ability of leukocytes from 3 uremic patients on dialysis to ingest and kill staphylococci. No significant abnormalities were detected in these 3 people. Hoffman [71] employed a bactericidal assay against *S. aureus* and *Escherichia coli* to study leukocyte function in 7 patients with renal failure. Six of the 7 had normal tests on repeated determinations. The patient who was abnormal was tested only once. Brogan [72] studied leukocyte function in 12 uremic patients in whom blood-urea levels ranged from 122 to 440 mg/100 ml. Morphologically, living polymorphs from patients with renal failure seemed to spread on glass slides more than control leukocytes. Cytoplasmic granules were more prominent and vacuoles were more common. Serum *independent* phagocytosis was significantly less in azotemic leukocytes than in normal cells. Ultrafiltrates of uremic or normal sera had no effect on the assay, indicating that no low-molecular weight toxic substances were likely present. Serum *dependent* phagocytosis was within normal limits and the addition of ultrafiltrates of uremic sera had no effect on either normal or uremic cells. The average concentration of salmonella endotoxin required to suppress the phagocytic activity of uremic leukocytes, however, was significantly less than that required to produce a similar suppression in normal cells. The finding suggests that uremic leukocytes may be more sensitive to the effects of endotoxin than cells from individuals with normal renal function.

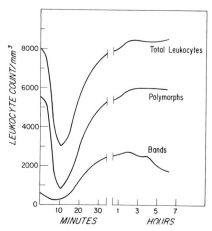

Fig. 3. Changes in leukocyte counts during initiation of hemodialysis. Fall in total leukocytes is due primarily to a marked reduction in polymorphs within the first few minutes after dialysis initiation. During the next hour, leukocytes tend to return toward normal and may rebound above normal.

Little is known of the effect of hemodialytic therapy on leukocyte function. However, a profound neutropenia occurs immediately following the start of hemodialysis [73-76]. Figure 3 illustrates the events that take place. Total leukocyte count begins to fall abruptly within the first 1 to 4 minutes after the first traces of blood are returned to the patient from the dialyzer. Total polymorphonuclear leukocyte count falls to reach a low of approximately 20 percent of the original value within the first 10 to 20 minutes. Then band forms rapidly increase and total leukocyte count is nearly normal after approximately 1 hour. Total leukocyte count then may [75,76] or may not [73,74] rebound above predialysis values. The phenomenon has been shown to occur with twin-coil, hollow fiber, and Kiil-type dialyzers [74] and is not attended by fever, chills, or other signs of endotoxemia.

The cause of this neutropenia is unknown but may be related to stagnation of blood within the dialyzer [76]. Leukocyte kinetic studies [75] have suggested that there is an immediate but perhaps temporary sequestration of functional leukocytes within the patient. With the fall in total leukocyte count, the specific activity of labeled leukocytes also falls. During recovery there may be some increase in specific activity of circulating cells. In 3 out of 5 patients studied in this fashion [75], specific activity returned to the expected values, indicating that almost all of the trapped leukocytes had returned to the general circulation. In 2 of 5 patients, it appeared that approximately one-fourth of the original circulating leukocytes may have been destroyed. The studies of Toren et al [77] have suggested that the leukocytes may be trapped within the pulmonary bed.

The stresses of pressure and shear during extracorporeal circulation may well effect the function of leukocytes. Kusserow and Larrow [78] found reduced phagocytic ability in leukocytes harvested from blood pumped in an extracorporeal circuit when compared to appropriate control samples. In these tests performed in an in vitro recirculating circuit, the degree of reduction in phagocytic index seemed to correlate with blood trauma as indicated by increases in plasma-free hemoglobin. Further studies by these investigators [79] demonstrated reduced oxygen comsumption in leukocytes that had been exposed to blood pumping in an in vitro perfusion circuit when compared to matched controls. Morphologic examination of the pumped cells revealed nuclear abnormalities and cytoplasmic changes described as a raggedness of cell contour. As with the erythrocyte, blood pumping may inflict damage upon leukocytes insufficient to cause outright destruction but which nonetheless causes significant metabolic derangements.

PLATELETS AND HEMOSTASIS

In the early 1900's Riesman [80] recognized bleeding as a complication of uremia and concluded that it may be caused by retained toxic factors. Current theory supports his thesis and recent work has led to the identification of such a substance [81].

Thrombocytopenia is commonly associated with chronic renal failure and may be observed in 30 to 40 percent of cases. When present it is usually mild, however [82,83], and adequate hemodialysis tends to restore platelet counts toward normal [83]. Normal clinical hemostasis may be observed in individuals with modestly reduced platelet counts while severe bleeding may be seen in patients whose platelet counts are quite normal. It is now generally believed that the primary thophysiology of uremic bleeding involves certain qualitative platelet aonormalities rather than a reduction in the absolute number of circulating platelets [82].

Lewis and colleagues [84] found that uremic platelets failed to improve the prothrombin consumption of normal platelet-poor plasma to the same extent as normal platelets. The defect was present in patients with normal bleeding times and negative tourniquet tests. Cahalane and associates [85] noted that incubation of a platelet extract in uremic plasma resulted in a greater loss of platelet factor 3 activity than incubation in normal plasma. The authors suggested that some metabolite retained in uremia inactivates platelet factor 3 in vivo. This interaction would then contribute to the bleeding manifestations that attend uremia.

Von Kaulla et al [86] also performed platelet function studies on untreated uremic patients, patients undergoing hemodialysis, and individuals after renal homotransplantation. They noted impaired platelet function with reduced thrombin generation and prothrombin consumption. Hemodialysis improved but did not always correct the abnormalities. In contrast, renal transplantation restored normal hemostasis and the improvement seemed to parallel renal function. They also concluded that some substance in uremic plasma may inhibit platelet function. Stewart and Castaldi [83] reported their observations on 17 patients, prior to and after dialysis, and demonstrated a number of qualitative platelet abnormalities including prolonged bleeding time, impaired platelet adhesiveness, impaired platelet aggregation, and abnormal platelet factor 3 availability. Adequate peritoneal dialysis improved all of the abnormalities. These investigators were unable to reproduce the platelet defect by the in vitro addition of urea, dextrose, mannitol, creatinine, urate, or phosphate or by changes of pH or osmolarity of the medium within the range that might be encountered in uremic individuals.

Rabiner and Hrodek [87] studied platelet factor 3 availability in 55 patients with uremia. Celite was used to activate platelet factor 3 release. In addition, platelet factor 3 content was studied by determining platelet factor 3 activity after disruption by freeze-thawing. Approximately three-fourths of patients exhibited abnormal activation. Platelet factor 3 content was abnormal in approximately one-third of patients. They concluded that the majority of uremic individuals have only defective release of the factor, but some may have both abnormal release and low content of platelet factor 3. Platelet factor 3 release returned to normal or was significantly improved within 24 to 48 hours after either peritoneal or hemodialysis.

Until recently, investigations for potential platelet toxins proved unrewarding. Urea was first considered an offending toxin. The addition of urea to normal platelets does not induce a functional defect [83], and no correlation between platelet factor 3 activity and blood urea levels has been demonstrated [87]. Nonetheless, Eknoyan and co-workers [88] showed a significant, inverse correlation between serum urea and creatinine levels and platelet adhesiveness. These findings alone do not necessarily imply that urea or creatinine per se is the offending agent because some substance with which urea and creatinine are covariates could well be responsible. They artificially induced azotemia in 10 normal volunteers who ingested 2 to 3 gm/kg body weight of urea at hourly intervals. Serum urea nitrogen levels of 60 to 120 mg/100 ml were maintained for 24 hours in some subjects. This treatment induced prolonged bleeding time in 5 individuals and decreased platelet adhesiveness to pathologic levels in 8. Again, these findings do not necessarily implicate urea in and of itself. Some compound which may increase in the serum as a result of *oral* urea loading may well be the responsible toxin. For instance Castaldi was unable to produce any detectable abnormality in platelet function by the *intravenous* infusion of urea into 2 normal subjects [89].

Guanidinosuccinic acid has been shown by Horowitz and associates [81] to be present in the serum of uremic individuals. Serum concentrations of this compound reach sufficient levels to inhibit adenosine diphosphate induced platelet factor 3 activation. Serum guanidinosuccinic acid levels and inhibition of platelet factor 3 activation tend to decrease in parallel in uremic patients who undergo dialysis. Exposure to guanidinosuccinic acid makes the dense tubular system of normal platelets prominent and tends to inhibit the normal morphologic changes that occur upon exposure to adenosine diphosphate. Of general and possibly therapeutic interest, the authors demonstrated acetylsalicylic acid to be as effective as guanidinosuccinic acid in inhibiting both platelet factor 3 activation and platelet aggregation.

The metabolic pathways by which guanidinosuccinic acid is generated have not been completely elucidated. It seems likely, however, that the compound is a product of arginine metabolism [90]. As such, ammonia or protein loading may well be expected to stimulate production of this compound and elevations of creatinine and urea might correlate with increased levels of guanidinosuccinic acid.

Phenolic compounds have also been implicated in the thrombocytopathy that attends chronic renal failure [91]. Pre-incubation of platelets with either phenol or parahydroxyphenylacetic acid produces significant inhibition of platelet factor 3 release. The concentrations of parahydroxyphenlacetic acid prevalent in uremic serum are sufficient to induce inhibition of platelet factor 3 release and platelet aggregation in vivo. No correlation between plasma levels of phenol and platelet factor 3 activity was demonstrated in this study. A significant correlation between plasma phenolic acid levels and platelet factor 3 was observed, however. As expected, plasma levels of both phenol and phenolic acid fall with hemodialysis. The mechanism by which these compounds may interfere with platelet function is not known and the relative roles of guanidinosuccinic acid and the phenols is uncertain.

It is generally held that hemodialysis improves platelet function. Nonetheless, preliminary observations have been presented [9] suggesting that in some patients hemodialysis may produce a relative deficiency syndrome which in turn causes impaired platelet function. Patients undergoing chronic hemodialysis were studied utilizing either high or low dialysate flow rates [92]. Low dialysate flow rate tends to relatively inhibit the removal of lower molecular weight compounds. Nonetheless, when low dialysate flow therapy was instituted, bleeding time shortened and tests of platelet adhesion improved in 4 patients. Theoretically, low flow inhibited the removal of some low molecular weight substance required for normal platelet function. These observations require confirmation.

The kinetics of platelets have been studied in extracorporeal blood circuits [93]. The behavior of chromium-labeled platelets was studied in experimental animals during extracorporeal circulation through membrane oxygenators, with and without the oxygenator in the circuit. Platelet counts and blood radioactivity fell promptly to approximately 60 percent of control values. Values tended to remain low, only to rise promptly upon termination of extracorporeal circulation. Both total platelet count and blood radioactivity rose upon completion of the procedure, indicating that sequestered platelets had returned to the circulation. Autopsy studies immediately after extracorporeal circulation revealed very little radioactivity in the lungs or kidneys, while significant radioactivity was present in the liver. The data suggest that some platelets are irreversibly lost during extracorporeal circulation. Nonetheless, there appears to be significant platelet sequestration which occurs primarily in the liver and is reversible. Although these studies may not be, strictly speaking, comparable to the events that transpire during hemodialysis, the similarity to the leukocyte alterations that attend hemodialysis is striking.

REFERENCES

1. Kasonen, A., Kalliomaki, J.L.: Correlation of some kidney function tests with hemoglobin in chronic nephropathies. Acta Med Scand 158:213, 1957.
2. Kaye, M.: The anemia associated with renal disease. J Lab Clin Med 52:82, 1958.
3. Callan, I.R., Limarzi, L.R.: Blood and bone marrow studies in renal disease. Am J Clin Pathol 20:3, 1950.
4. Schwartz, S.O., Motto, S.A.: The diagnostic significance of "Burr" red blood cells. Am J Med Sci 218:563, 1949.

5. Aherne, W.A.: The "Burr" red cell and azotemia. J Clin Pathol 10:252, 1957.
6. Hampers, C.L., Streiff, R., Nathan, D., et al: Megaloblastic hematopoiesis in uremia and in patients on long-term hemodialysis. N Engl J Med 276:35, 1967.
7. Whitehead, V.M., Comty, C.H., Posen, G.A., et al: Homeostasis of folic acid in patients undergoing maintenance hemodialysis. N Engl J Med 279:970, 1968.
8. Erslev, A.: Humoral regulation of red cell production. Blood 8:349, 1953.
9. Jacobson, L.O., Goldwasser, E., Fried, W., et al: Role of the kidney in erythropoiesis. Nature [New Biol] 179:633, 1957.
10. Naets, J.P.: The role of the kidney in erythropoiesis. J Clin Invest 39:102, 1960.
11. Gordon, A.S.: The current status of erythropoietin. Br J Haematol 21:611, 1971.
12. Peschle, C., Sasso, G.F., Rappaport, I.A., et al Erythropoietin production in nephrectomized rats: Possible role of the renal erythropoietic factor. J Lab Clin Med 79:950, 1972.
13. Nathan, D.G., Schupak, E., Stohlman, F., et al: Erythropoiesis in anephric man. J Clin Invest 43:2158, 1964.
14. Naets, J.P., Wittek, M., Toussaint, C., et al: Erythropoiesis in renal insufficiency and in anephric man. Ann N Y Acad Sci 149:143, 1968.
15. Naets, J.P., Wittek, M.: Presence of erythropoietin in the plasma of one anephric patient. Blood 31:249, 1968.
16. Kominami, N., Lowrie, E.G., Ianhez, L.E., et al: The effect of total nephrectomy on hematopoiesis in patients undergoing chronic hemodialysis. J Lab Clin Med 78:524, 1971.
17. Naets, J.P., Heuse, A.F.: Measurement of erythropoietic stimulating factor in anemic patients with or without renal disease. J Lab Clin Med 60:365, 1962.
18. Gallagher, N.I., McCarthy, J.M., Lange, R.D.: Observations on erythropoietic-stimulating factor (ESF) in the plasma of uremic and nonuremic anemic patients. Ann Intern Med 52:1201, 1960.
19. Reismann, K.R., Nomura, T., Gunn, R.W., et al: Erythropoietic response to anemia or erythropoietin injection in uremic rats with or without functioning renal tissue. Blood 16:1411, 1960.
20. Mann, D.L., Donati, R.M., Gallagher, N.I.: Erythropoietin assay and ferrokinetic measurements in anemic uremic patients. JAMA 194:1321, 1965.
21. Denny, W.F., Flanigan, W.J., Zukoski, C.: Serial erythropoietin studies in patients undergoing renal homotransplantation. J Lab Clin Med 67:386, 1966.
22. Takasuci, M., Imura, S.: Iron absorption and utilization in chronic nephritis. Am J Med Sci 254:56, 1967.
23. Finch, C.A., Deubeleiss, J., Cook, J., et al: Ferrokinetics in man. Medicine (Baltimore) 49:17, 1970.

24. Cook, J.D., Marsaglia, G., Eschbach, J.W., et al: Ferrokinetics: A biologic model for plasma iron exchange in man. J Clin Invest 49:197, 1970.
25. DesForges, J.F., Dawson, J.P.: The anemia of renal failure. Arch Intern Med 101:326, 1958.
26. Joske, R.A., McAlister, J.M., Prankerd, T.A.J.: Isotope investigations of red cell production and destruction in chronic renal disease. Clin Sci 15:511, 1956.
27. Loge, J.P., Lange, R.D., Moore, C.V.: Characterization of the anemia associated with chronic renal insufficiency. Am J Med 24:4, 1958.
28. Eschbach, J.W., Funk, D., Adamson, J., et al: Erythropoiesis in patients with renal failure undergoing chronic dialysis. N Engl J Med 276:653, 1967.
29. Van Ypersele de Strihou, C., Stragier, A.: Effect of bilateral nephrectomy on transfusion requirements of patients undergoing chronic dialysis. Lancet 2:705, 1969.
30. Markson, J.L., Rennie, J.B.: The anaemia of chronic renal insufficiency. Scott Med J 1:320, 1956.
31. Berman, L., Powsner, E.R.: Review of methods for studying maturation of human erythroblasts in vitro: Evaluation of a new method of culture of cell suspensions in a clot-free medium. Blood 14:1194, 1959.
32. Thorup, O.A., Strole, W.E., Leavell, B.S.: The rate of removal of iron from culture medium by human bone marrow suspension. J Lab Clin Med 32:266, 1958.
33. Erslev, A.J., Hughes, J.R.: The influence of environment on iron incorporation and mitotic division in a suspension of normal bone marrow. Br J Haematol 6:414, 1960.
34. Markson, J.L., Moore, J.M.: The anaemia of chronic renal insufficiency: Autoradiographic studies in normoblasts cultured in uraemic serum. Br J Haematol 8:414, 1962.
35. Henkin, R.I., Levine, N.D., Sussman, H.H., et al: Evidence for the presence of substances toxic for HeLa cells in the serum and in the dialysis fluid of patients with glomerulonephritis. J Lab Clin Med 64:79, 1964.
36. Quadracci, L.J., Cambi, V., Christopher, T.G., et al: Assay of serum abnormalities in uremic and dialysis patients: Evidence for depletion of vital substances in hemodialysis. Trans Am Soc Artif Intern Organs 17:96, 1971.
37. Rachmilewitz, M.: Effect of uremic serum and urine on growth of fibroblasts in vitro. Arch Intern Med 67:1132, 1941.
38. Kurtides, E.S., Rambach, W.A., Alt, H.L., et al: Effect of hemodialysis on erythrokinetics in anemia of uremia. J Lab Clin Med 63:469, 1964.
39. DeGowin, R.L., Lavender, A.R., Forland, M., et al: Erythropoiesis and erythropoietin in patients with chronic renal failure treated with hemodialysis and testosterone. Ann Intern Med 72:913, 1970.
40. Richardson, J.R., Weinstein, M.B.: Erythropoietic response of dialyzed patients to testosterone administration. Ann Intern Med 73:403, 1970.

41. Mirand, E.A., Murphy, G.P., Steeves, R.A., et al: Erythropoietic activity in anephric, allotransplanted, unilaterally nephrectomized and intact man. J Lab Clin Med 73:121, 1969.
42. Shaldon, S., Patyna, W., Kaltwasser, P., et al: The use of testosterone in bilaterally nephrectomized patients. Trans Am Soc Artif Intern Organs 17:104, 1971.
43. Wang, F., Fried, W.: Renal and extrarenal erythropoietin production in male and female rats of various ages. J Lab Clin Med 79:181, 1972.
44. Resan, T.K., Shahidi, N.T., Korst, D.R.: The effect of phenobarbital on testosterone-induced erythropoiesis. J Lab Clin Med 79:187, 1972.
45. Kennedy, A.C.: Blood loss in regular dialysis. Abstract of Plenary Sessions and Symposia, Fifth International Congress of Nephrology, Oct, 1972, p 62.
46. Comty, C.M., McDade, D., Kaye, M.: Anemia and iron requirements of patients treated by maintenance hemodialysis. Trans Am Soc Artif Intern Organs 14:426, 1968.
47. Emerson, C.D.: The pathogenesis of anemia in acute glomerulonephritis: estimates of blood destruction and production in a case receiving massive transfusions. Blood 3:363, 1948.
48. Ragen, P.A., Hagedorn, A.B., Owen, C.A.: Radioisotopic study of anemia in chronic renal disease. Arch Intern Med 105:518, 1960.
49. Giovannetti, S., Balestri, P.L., Cioni, L.: Spontaneous in vitro auto-haemolysis of blood from chronic uraemic patients. Clin Sci 29:407, 1965.
50. Welt, L.G., Sachs, J.R., McManus, T.J.: Anion transport defect in erythrocytes from uremic patients. Trans Assoc Am Physicians 77: 169, 1964.
51. Cole, C.H., Balfe, J.W., Welt, L.G.: Induction of a oubian-sensitive ATPase defect by uremic plasma. Trans Assoc Am Physicians 81:213, 1968.
52. Welt, L., Smith, E., Dunn, M., et al: Membrane transport defect; The sick cell. Trans Assoc Am Physicians 80:217, 1967.
53. Hyde, S.E., Sadler, J.: Red blood cell destruction in hemodialysis. Trans Am Soc Artif Intern Organs 15:50, 1969.
54. Indeglia, R.A., Shea, M., Forstram, R., et al: Influence of mechanical factors on erythrocyte sublethal damage. Trans Am Soc Artif Intern Organs 14:264, 1968.
55. Indeglia, R., Bernstein, E.: Selective lipid loss following mechanical erythrocyte damage. Trans Am Soc Artif Intern Organs 16:37, 1970.
56. Bernstein, E.: Erythrocyte metabolism following surface induced injury. Trans Am Soc Artif Intern Organs 17:386, 1971.
57. Sutra, S.P., Croce, P., Mehrjardi, M.: Hemolysis and subhemolytic alteration of human RBC induced by turbulent shearflow. Trans Am Soc Artif Intern Organs 18:335, 1972.
58. Yawata, Y., Kjellstrand, C., Buselmeier, T., et al: Hemolysis in dialyzed patients: Tap water induced red blood cell metabolic deficiency. Trans Am Soc Artif Intern Organs 18:301, 1972.

59. Manzier, A.D., Schreiner, A.W.: Copper-induced acute hemolytic anemia; A new complication of hemodialysis. Ann Intern Med 73:409, 1970.

60. Carlson, D.J., Shapiro, F.L.: Methemoglobinemia from well water nitrates: a complication of home hemodialysis. Ann Intern Med 73:757, 1970.

61. Bischel, M.D., Neiman, R.W., Berne, T.V., et al: The elimination by splenectomy of blood transfusion requirements, leukopaenia and thrombocytopaenia in the patient on RDT. Proc Europ Dial Transplt Assoc 8:81, 1971.

62. Hartley, L.C.J., Innis, M.D., Morgan, T.O., et al: Splenectomy for anaemia in patients on regular haemodialysis. Lancet 2:1343, 1971.

63. Blendis, L.M., Clarke, M.D., Williams, R.: Effect of splenectomy on the haemodilutional anaemia of splenomegaly. Lancet 1:795, 1969.

64. Finch, C.A., Lenfant, C.: Oxygen transport in man. N Engl J Med 286: 407, 1972.

65. Hurt, G.A., Chanutin, A.: Organic phosphate compounds of erythrocytes from individuals with uremia. J Lab Clin Med 64:675, 1964.

66. Lichtman, M.A., Miller, D.R.: Erythrocyte glycolysis, 2, 3-diphosphoglycerate and adenosine triphosphate concentration in uremic subjects: Relationship to extracellular phosphate concentration. J Lab Clin Med 76:267, 1970.

67. Mitchell, T.R., Pegrum, G.D.: The oxygen affinity of haemoglobin in chronic renal failure. Br J Haemotol 21:463, 1971.

68. Parker, J.P., Beirne, G.J., Desai, J.N., et al: Androgen-induced increase in red-cell, 2, 3-diphosphoglycerate. N Engl J Med 287:381, 1972.

69. Siddiqui, J., Freeburger, R., Freeman, R.M.: Folic acid, hypersegmented polymorphonuclear leukocytes and the uremic syndrome. Am J Clin Nutr 23:11, 1970.

70. Alexander, J., Hegg, M., Altemeier, W.: Neutrophil function in selected surgical disorders. Ann Surg 168:447, 1968.

71. Hoffman, T.A.: Personal communication.

72. Brogan, T.D.: Phagocytosis by polymorphonuclear leucocytes from patients with renal failure. Br Med J 3:596, 1967.

73. Kaplow, L., Goffinet, J.: Profound neutropenia during the early phase of hemodialysis. JAMA 203:1135, 1968.

74. Gral, T., Schroth, P., DePalma, J., et al: Leukocyte dynamics with three types of dialyzers. Trans Am Soc Artif Intern Organs 15:45, 1969.

75. Brubaker, L., Nolph, K.: Mechanisms of recovery from neutropenia induced by hemodialysis. Blood 38:623, 1972.

76. Brubaker, L., Jensen, D., Johnson, C., et al: Kinetics of stagnation-induced neutropenia during hemodialysis. Trans Am Soc Artif Intern Organs 18:305, 1972.

77. Toren, M., Goffinet, J., Kaplow, L.: Pulmonary bed sequestration of neutrophils during hemodialysis. Blood 36:337, 1970.

78. Kussenow, B., Larrow, R.: Studies of leukocyte response to prolonged blood pumping—effects upon phagocytic capability and total white cell count. Trans Am Soc Artif Intern Organs 14:261, 1968.
79. Kussenow, B., Larrow, R., Nichols, J.: Metabolic and morphologic alterations in leukocytes following prolonged blood pumping. Trans Am Soc Artif Intern Organs 15:40, 1969.
80. Riesman, D.: Hemorrhages in the course of Bright's disease with especial reference to the occurrence of a hemorrhagic diathesis of nephritic origin. Am J Med Sci 134:709, 1907.
81. Horowitz, H., Stein, J., Cohen, B., et al: Further studies on the platelet-inhibitory effect of guanidinosuccinic acid and its role in uremic bleeding. Am J Med 49:336, 1970.
82. Rabner, S.F.: Uremic bleeding, in Spaet T. (ed): Progress in hemostasis and thrombosis, vol. 1. New York, Grune & Stratton, 1971, p 233.
83. Stewart, J.H., Castaldi, P.A.: Uraemic bleeding: A reversible platelet defect corrected by dialysis. Q J Med 36:409, 1967.
84. Lewis, J., Zucker, M., Ferguson, J.: Bleeding tendency in uremia. Blood 11:1073, 1956.
85. Cahalane, S., Johnson, S., Monto, S., et al: Acquited thrombocytopathy. Observations on the coagulation defects in uremia. Am J Clin Pathol 30:507, 1958.
86. Von Kaulla, K.N., Von Kaulla, E., Wasantapruck, S., et al: Blood coagulation in uremic patients before and after hemodialysis and transplantation of the kidney. Arch Surg 92:184, 1966.
87. Rabiner, S.F., Hrodek, O.: Platelet factor 3 in normal subjects and patients with renal failure. J Clin Invest 47:901, 1968.
88. Eknoyan, G., Wacksman, J., Glueck, H., et al: Platelet function in renal failure. N Engl J Med 280:677, 1969.
89. Castaldi, P., Rozenberg, M.D., Stewart, J.H.: Bleeding disorder of uraemic: qualitative platelet defect. Lancet 2:66, 1966.
90. Cohen, B.: Guanidinosuccinic acid in uremia. Arch Intern Med 7:846, 1970.
91. Rabiner, S.F., Molinas, F.: The role of phenol and phenolic acids on the thrombocytopathy and defective platelet aggregation of patients with renal failure. Am J Med 49:346, 1970.
92. Christopher, T., Cambi, V., Harker, L., et al: A Study of Hemodialysis with lowered dialysate flow rate. Trans Am Soc Artif Intern Organs 17:92, 1971.
93. DeLeval, M., Hill, D., Mielke, H., et al: Platelet kinetics during extra-corporeal circulation. Trans Am Soc Artif Intern Organs 18:355, 1972.

7

The Gastrointestinal System

The gastrointestinal system plays an important role in the symptomatology of patients with chronic renal failure. Presenting symptoms are often metallic taste, anorexia, and/or nausea and vomiting. These symptoms may complicate the uremic patient's course by inducing volume depletion, vitamin deficiency and/or negative nitrogen balance. There is some misunderstanding concerning the benefits of a low-protein diet in this group of patients. Although blood urea nitrogen and other protein metabolites may be lowered, the benefit of such a diet appears to be only in alleviating nausea and vomiting—no evidence suggests that the diet that corrects other underlying uremia symptoms. For some patients, these less palatable diets may be more undesirable than the symptoms they prevent. If the uremic patient has no gastrointestinal symptoms and hemodialysis is in the offing for other reasons, we feel that protein in the diet should not be severely restricted and should be titrated to the gastrointestinal symptoms. This is particularly important in children, whose growth rates may be adversely affected by negative nitrogen balance. Sodium and, more importantly, potassium restriction must be continued.

In the terminal stages of uremia, patients may present with stomatitis, esophagitis, gastritis, duodenitis, ileitis, or colitis. In an extensive postmortem review of the digestive tract in uremia Jaffe and Lain [1] found 27.1 percent of patients with mucosal edema, 52.9 percent with hemorrhages in the mucosa, and 19.8 percent with psuedomembranous and ulcerative lesions. The abnormalities, seen from the lower esophagus to the colon, predominated in the ileum and colon, presumably because of high bacterial growth rates in these areas. These authors concluded, however, that the ulcerative lesions were secondary to mucosal edema and hemorrhages that occurred as a result of circulatory disturbances.

Most or all of the gastrointestinal symptoms in uremic patients will rapidly clear with a course of hemodialysis. If nausea and vomiting continue during the hemodialysis procedure, they are likely related to other factors such as hypovolemia and hypotension, which usually occur either early in the procedure as the patient is "bled" into the dialyzer or late in the dialysis when intravascular volume is maximally depleted. Vomiting may occur during or immediately after the onset of hypotension and responds promptly to volume repletion. However, blood pressure taken after emesis may be elevated and therefore cause misleading therapeutic implications. One must be well trained, particularly in the home dialysis situation, in handling patients in this condition. Aspiration must be prevented while the blood pressure is monitored, saline is administered, and the pump speed is adjusted. Having the patient assume the Trendelenburg position may help minimize symptoms during periods of low blood pressure. Nausea and vomiting may occur at times other than during the dialysis procedure, frequently without identifiable cause. Although antiemetic drugs are usually of little help, prochlorperazine and Tigan may give some relief to the rare patient who complains of chronic nausea and vomiting. However, one must be aware of the extrapyramidal side effects of the phenothiazin drugs in uremic patients.

Gastrointestinal hemorrhage in the severely uremic patient will frequently abate with hemodialysis. Whether this is due to correction of an altered clotting mechanism or removal of some toxic metabolite or both is not clear. When there is evidence of gastrointestinal bleeding, the patient being initiated on hemodialysis should obviously receive regional heparinization. This is only necessary for one or two hemodialyses, however, and the gastrointestinal bleeding usually ceases. The occurrence of gastrointestinal hemorrhage in the well-dialyzed patient implies nonuremic pathology and demands further investigation of the gastrointestinal tract. Bailey et al [2] have demonstrated an increased incidence of hiatus hernia in uremic patients, particularly those with polycystic kidney disease. Hiatus hernia may result in esophagitis with bleeding. There is also an increased incidence of colonic diverticuli in uremic patients [2]. Again, this is most prominently seen in patients with polycystic kidney disease. Diverticulosis may be complicated by diverticulitis and result in an increased incidence of lower GI bleeding and colonic rupture. With increasing age of patients accepted for hemodialysis, the population at risk will also have a significant incidence of malignancy of the GI tract (unrelated to uremia), which must be considered in individuals with continued gastrointestinal blood loss.

Peptic ulcer disease in the stomach and duodenum has been suggested to be more common in patients with chronic renal failure. Early papers [3-5] reporting results of long-term dialysis described peptic ulceration occurring in approximately 20 percent of patients. Hampers and Schupak [6] reported an incidence of 11 percent and pointed out that this may not be greater than the incidence in the population at large. Other reports from smaller series, however, continue to document a higher incidence of peptic ulcer disease [7]. We have appreciated that a number of patients with renal failure are referred with a diagnosis of peptic ulcer disease based on suggestive rather than definitive evidence. The similarity of uremic gastroduodenal disease and nonuremic peptic ulcer disease must be recognized. In an autopsy series of uremic patients, Moynihan [8] found that the duodenal ulcers examined could not be pathologically distinguished from peptic ulcers.

One of the major difficulties in the diagnosis of peptic ulcer in these uremic patients is the sometimes confusing radiologic appearance of the gastrointestinal tract. Wiener, Vertes, and Shapiro [9], in a study of 48 uremic patients, found three abnormal upper gastrointestinal patterns—the first, "wet stomach," was characterized by prominent gastric folds and decreased gastric peristalsis with a prolonged emptying time. In his radiology textbook, Meschan [10] also points out the frequent finding of gastric atony in uremic patients. Although this may be due to atropic or chronic gastritis, it could also be the result of neuropathy of the autonomic nervous system, as has been suggested previously [11-13]. The second abnormal GI pattern discussed by Wiener et al [9] is prominent, enlarged duodenal folds that are linear and irregular. The third pattern is enlarged folds in the descending duodenum. Wiener and his associates point out the possibility of erroneous diagnosis of bulbar deformity in these patients.

In another review of upper gastrointestinal radiographic examinations, Bailey et al [2] report on 85 uremic patients *selected* for radiographic examinations because of gastrointestinal symptoms. In their series 28 percent had hiatal hernia and 21 percent had duodenal ulcer, while 44 percent had mucosal edema of the stomach or duodenum. Van den Bogaert et al [14] in a study of 20 renal patients also found a high incidence of hypertrophic or edematous mucosa and gastric fluid retention. King et al [15] in their study of 18 uremic patients found 8 with abnormal x-rays of the small bowel due to edema or hemorrhage in the mucosa. Figure 1 is an example of the gastric mucosal edema and duodenal bulb deformity seen in uremia that may be confused with peptic ulcer disease and, as illustrated, improves with hemodialysis. The altered radiographic picture in uremic patients therefore necessitates that the diagnosis of peptic ulcer disease in either the stomach or duodenum be deferred until adequate hemodialysis has been instituted and the studies repeated. We have not found the incidence of peptic ulcer disease to be greater in dialyzed uremic patients than in the general population.

The x-ray findings of duodenitis are similar to those seen in chronic pancreatitis. Interestingly 9 of the patients in the series of Wiener [9] were suspected of having pancreatitis. This was subsequently proven in 6 at postmortem examination. Elevated serum amylase values frequently noted in uremic patients are thought to be secondary to decreased urinary excretion [16]. Usually the hyperamylasemia associated with chronic renal failure is mild to moderate (that is, less than 200 to 300 Somogyi units) and massive increases in amylase should suggest the presence of pancreatitis. It has been suggested that pancreatic function is further impaired by a decrease in bicarbonate in pancreatic secretion secondary to chronic acidosis [17]. This may play a role in the increased incidence of gastric disease in uremia patients. The similar x-ray pictures of the duodenum in patients with uremia and pancreatitis may be related to a combination of both diseases. However, in our program postmortem examination or laporatomy documentation of pancreatitis has not occurred frequently.

The role of gastric acid secretion in the development of gastroduodenal lesions in uremia has been evaluated by a number of investigators. Lieber and Lefevre [18] found low free and total acid concentrations in uremic subjects and felt the decreased gastric acidity was the result of neutralization with high gastric ammonia. On the other hand, Mossberg et al [19] in a study of uremic patients did not find lowered stomach acid and there was no correlation between ammonia and gastric acidity. Goldstein et al [20], Gingell et al [21], Wiener et al [9], and Hampers and Schupak [22] all found normal acid secretion on stimulation studies, and only Ventkateswaren [23] and Fillastre et al [24] found hyperacidic secretion. In none of these studies was a relationship between gastric and duodenal lesions and gastric acidity identified. Gastric acid production has been reported to increase with hypercalcemia [20,25]; however, this does not usually apply to the uremic patient unless hypercalcemia is iatrogenically produced. Ward et al [26] reported increase in basal acid output in patients with *primary* hyperparathyroidism, and Barreras and Donaldson [27]

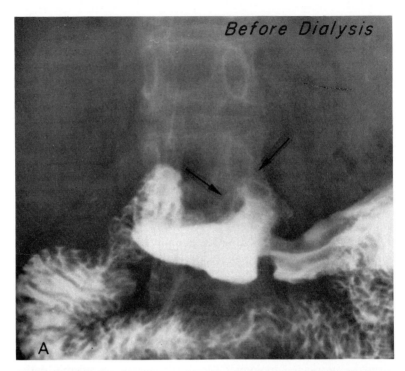

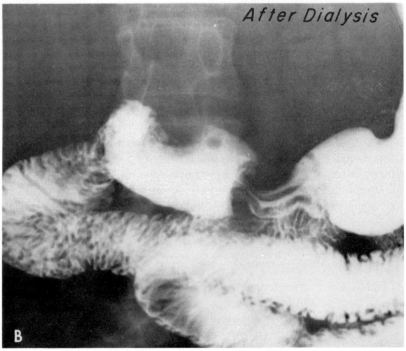

140

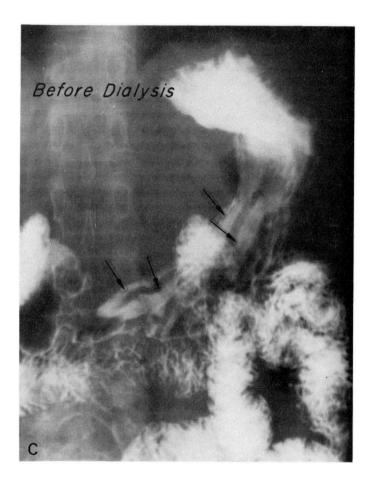

Fig. 1. Upper gastrointestinal series in a uremic female before and after initiation of hemodialysis. Study was initially performed for nausea and vomiting without a peptic ulcer history. Note thickened edematous gastric folds and duodenal bulb deformity. After 2 weeks of hemodialysis without other treatment, upper gastrointestinal x-ray revealed marked reduction of mucosal edema with improvement in apparent duodenal deformity. *(A)* and *(C):* before dialysis; *(B)* and *(D):* after dialysis.

141

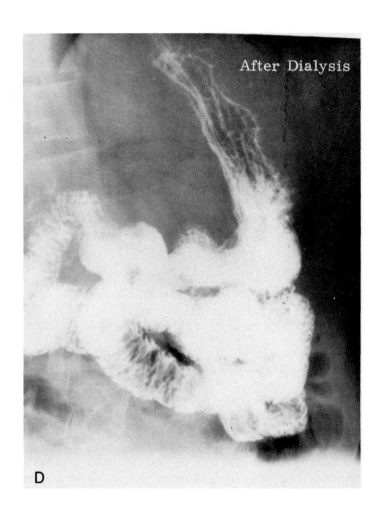

Fig. 1D. (Legend on preceding page.)

found that removal of a parathyroid adenoma in a patient with a high gastric acid output reduced the calcium and gastric output to normal. However, increased gastric acidity or ulcer disease specifically related to *secondary* hyperparathyroidism of uremia has not been demonstrated.

Gastrin levels determined by radioimmunoassay are elevated in uremic patients. Durkin et al [28] suggested that gastrin production was increased and demonstrated that, although the substance itself could be removed by peritoneal dialysis, there was no appreciable decrease in serum levels. In anephric patients Maxwell et al [29] found elevated gastrin levels that returned to normal after successful transplantation. They suggested there was a reduction in the degradation of gastrin by diseased or absent kidneys. Korman et al [30] found elevated gastrin levels which correlated with the serum creatinine and did not decrease appreciably with hemodialysis. Their patients also regained normal gastrin levels after transplantation, again suggesting a defect in degradation. Reeder and Thompson [31], on the other hand, concluded that serum gastrin concentrations in uremic patients did not differ from those of normals and did not change with hemodialysis. In none of these studies has a relationship between hypergastrinemia, hyper- or hypogastric acidity, and gastric or duodenal lesions been demonstrated.

There have been several isolated reports of gastrointestinal bleeding in chronically dialyzed patients; however, the series are small and the true incidence is unknown. In their study of 48 patients, Wiener et al [9] mention gastrointestinal hemorrhage in 5 who, incidentially, had radiographic findings which were not different from the uremic population as a whole. Ventkateswaran et al [23] found 2 of 10 patients on chronic hemodialysis with peptic ulcers; however, the authors do not discuss the incidence of gastrointestinal hemorrhage. Lewicki et al [32] in a study of a mixed group of 285 dialysis and transplant patients found 51 requiring upper gastrointestinal series for symptoms. In the pretransplant group, only 5 GI series were performed to determine the cause of gastrointestinal bleeding. Penn et al [33] in a study of 184 transplant recipients found 4 with bleeding from peptic ulcers or gastritis *prior to* transplantation. Boner and Berry [7] reported 5 cases of gastrointestinal hemorrhage in a group of 14 chronic hemodialysis patients. In our dialysis patient population of more than 300, upper gastrointestinal hemorrhage is an unusual occurrence and, when present, usually has a definable etiology. The avoidance or judicious use of anticoagulants or other drugs such as acetylsalicyclic acid might be important in preventing or controlling gastrointestinal bleeding.

Recently it has been suggested that chronic dialysis patients anticipating renal transplantation should have thorough gastrointestinal evaluation, prophylactic gastrointestinal surgery should be considered if hyperacidity or definite disease is found. Gordon et al [34] observed gastrointestinal bleeding in 5 of their first 19 transplants; however, in a subsequent study of 56 pretransplant patients, they found abnormal upper gastrointestinal series in only 5 patients—3 with gastric ulcers, 1 with coarse duodenal folds, and only 1 with a chronic duodenal ulcer. The correlation between these lesions, G.I. bleeds, and hypo- or hypersecretion was not impressive and in our opinion does not warrant their conclusion that prophylactic gastrectomy should be considered in patients with abnormally high gastric secretion. Hadjiyannakis et al [35] found 15 of 139 transplant patients with upper gastrointestinal bleeding and perforation; however, only 2 had ulcer disease diagnosed prior to transplantation, and 1 of these had had prophylactic surgery. In 184 transplant patients, Penn et al [33] found 6 who had pretransplant gastrointestinal problems, and 4 of these patients had G.I. bleeding due either to peptic ulcer or gastritis. Twenty-two post-transplant patients has gastrointestinal complications—of these 2 had gastric ulcer perforations, 3 had gastritis, and only 3 had duodenal ulcers (1 of whom had prophylactic surgery before transplantation). Coleman et al [36] in 54 transplant patients found 6 with gastrointestinal hemorrhage, but found duodenal ulcers in only 2 patients. In these studies no relationship between pretransplant symptoms or x-ray findings was demonstrated with presence or absence of post-transplant pathology.

Before accepting a philosophy of prophylactic surgery, several points should be considered. First, the incidence of abnormal gastrointestinal series in uremic patients may lead to a false-positive diagnosis of peptic ulcer disease in the pretransplant group. This has been discussed above. Second, a causal relationship between corticosteroids and gastric ulcers has been suggested, and in a recent correspondence, Coleman et al [36] suggested that the gastric mucosal barrier is impaired due to use of steroids, and this may cause an increased incidence of gastritis or gastric ulcers. A relationship between steroids and duodenal ulcers, however, is less conclusive, as has been pointed out by Cooke [37]. Likewise, an association between previously diagnosed peptic ulcer disease and recurrent ulcer disease or gastrointestinal bleeding after the institution of corticosteroids has not been documented, although this is a distinct possibility. If the gastrointestinal lesion associated with corticosteroids is gastric rather than duodenal, one must question the rationale of prophylactic surgery which may further impede gastric emptying in uremic patients in whom it has been demonstrated to be delayed. Persistent gastric lesions, symptomatic disease, or uncontrollable bleeding should of course be handled as in other patients. Although gastrointestinal disease with bleeding may be one of the common complications in the post-transplant period, further documentation of the beneficial effects of *prophylactic* surgery must be demonstrated before chronic hemodialysis patients are routinely subjected to such operations. We currently perform subtotal gastrectomy, antrectomy, and vagotomy in chronic dialysis patients awaiting transplantation if there is documented evidence of previous gastrointestinal hemorrhage and persistent duodenal bulb changes which are felt not to be the result of uremia. Subsequent comparison of this group of patients to patients who have previously undergone transplantation with such lesions and without prophylactic surgery and to a population with known absence of gastroduodenal disease will help determine the advisability of the procedure. These data are currently unavailable.

Phosphate-binding aluminum antacid gels are used extensively in patients on chronic hemodialysis. This is discussed in the section on calcium metabolism (Chap. 9). The large doses of the antacids required may cause nausea and vomiting in some uremic patients, and the type of antacid may have to be altered. Although hyperaluminumemia has been reported [38] in patients on chronic hemodialysis ingesting such products, a specific detrimental effect of an increased serum aluminum level has not been found. Some antacid products contain magnesium and, especially in the presence of high magesium dialysate, hypermagnesemia may inadvertently develop. This may be life threatening and should be avoided. Antacids, along with ferrous gluconate or ferrous sulfate, may also cause constipation and bulk laxatives may be required along with this therapy.

Chronic constipation and fecal impaction should be avoided in dialyzed patients. Difficult bowel movements with straining of hard stools, digital deimpaction, and enemas may create a problem in patients who have recently undergone hemodialysis with heparinization. The possibility of rupturing of diverticuli should also be considered in the chronically constipated patient. Intramural hematomas of the gastrointestinal tract are not unusual and have been reported on a number of occasions [39,40]. In most case reports these have been secondary to the use of Coumadin or bishydroxycoumarin, but we have also noted heparin to be important in the development of intramural hematomas. One elderly patient developed an intraumural hematoma with sigmoid obstruction secondary to digital examination during hemodialysis; following deimpaction, another patient had a massive intramural hematoma that ruptured, leading to death; and a child developed an intramural hematoma with sigmoid obstruction as the result of trauma from an enema nozzle administered following dialysis. We witnessed an intramural hematoma in the esophagus in a patient who developed gradual dysphasia, with a barium swallow revealing an esophageal mass. This patient had been on Coumadin for persistent clotting of an arteriovenous shunt and her prothrombin time was abnormally prolonged. This history, along with the smooth indentation of the mass on x-ray, suggested that it was an intramural hematoma. With institution of regional heparinization and discontinuance of the Coumadin, the esophageal mass disappeared over a 3-week period (see Fig. 2). The occurrence of abdominal wall hematomas in dialysis patients has been reported by DeSanto and his co-workers [46]. They described 4 cases of hematoma in the rectus abdominus muscle in patients undergoing peritoneal or hemodialysis. We witnessed 1 patient with a gradually enlarging abdomen thought to be ascites but which,

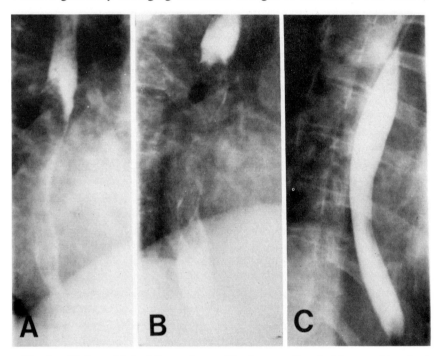

Fig. 2. Right and left oblique views of barium swallow in 34-year-old patient with sudden onset of dysphagia *(A* and *B)*. Treated with regional heparinization with relief of symptoms in 2 weeks and x-ray showing resolution of mass *(C)*.

following a four-quadrant abdominal tap, proved to be an intra-abdominal wall hematoma. The diagnosis can usually be made by paracentesis, although laparotomy may be necessary in some cases. The institution of regional heparinization is essential once the diagnosis is made.

Significant ascites, not uncommon in uremic patients, most often due to excessive extracellular volume and congestive heart failure, and with sufficient time it can be removed by aggressive ultrafiltration. The occurrence of persistent idiopathic ascites in chronically dialyzed patients not related to fluid excess has been reported [43-45]. We recently cared for 4 patients with ascites who underwent extensive diagnostic evaluation—multiple paracenteses with analysis of ascitic fluid, upper and lower gastrointestinal x-rays, lymphangiogram, arteriogram, splenoportagram, liver biopsy, cardiac catheterization, and, on one occasion, laparotomy. All results were negative. Ascites resolved in the first patient without change in the dialysis procedure. The second patient died from other causes and at postmortem examination no abdominal or gastrointestinal abnormality was found. The third patient underwent renal transplantation and, after normal renal function was resumed, the ascitic fluid disappeared. The final patient had an unusual but recognized cause for her ascites—she had inadvertently discontinued thyroid medication and over an 8-month period had become hypothyroid. Reinstitution of her thyroid medication alleviated the ascitic accumulation. The occurrence of unexplained ascites is rare in chronic dialysis patients, but when present complicates the dialysis and may respond only to successful renal transplantation.

Hepatic abnormalities in patients with chronic renal failure are common and require careful evaluation. Most of the literature on liver abnormalities in hemodialysis patients has justifiably been concerned with viral hepatitis and its hazard in dialysis units. Many patients on chronic hemodialysis have elevated serum glutamic oxaloacetic transaminase (SGOT) and serum glutamic pyruvic transaminase (SGPT) or lactic dehydrogenase (LDH), and the presumptive diagnosis of hepatitis is made [46,47]. A number of these patients, however, may have laboratory abnormalities as the result of disorders other than viral hepatitis. In many uremic patients, particularly before hemodialysis, there is increased extracellular volume and congestive heart failure with resultant chronic passive congestion of the liver. In most cases with this basic cause for altered liver function, the response to hemodialysis and ultrafiltration is prompt and impressive. In addition, dialysis patients are exposed to a number of potentially hepatotoxic drugs such as testosterone, oral estrogens, halothane, methyl fluorathane, Butazolidin, griseofulvin, and oxacillin. Drug-induced liver disease must therefore always be considered.

Hemodialysis patients may have pneumonia, sepsis, or shock with secondary toxic hepatic changes, as well as the so-called postoperative jaundice [48]. Obscure bacterial, fungal, and protozoal liver infections are rare in this country, but must be remembered as a possibility in hemodialysis patients. Concomitant diseases, such as carcinoma, hemochromatosis, polycystic liver disease, sarcoidosis, or collagen diseases may also adversely affect the liver. Furthermore, extrahepatic biliary obstruction must be ruled out as in any patient with jaundice. Bergman et al [49] feel there is a "nonspecific" hepatitis in chronic dialysis patients. Although this may be true, viral hepatitis with a wide spectrum of severity is probably the most common cause of abnormal liver function in this population.

Elevations of SGOT, SGPT, and LDH are nonspecific and in most cases do not aid the physician in the differential diagnosis. The presence of an abnormally high alkaline phosphatase has also generally not been helpful because of the presence of concurrent bone disease. The use of heat-stabilized alkaline phosphatase may prove more informative in this regard. Bilirubin elevations are unusual, occur late, and indicate a more advanced involvement. A liver scan may help rule out mass lesions. Since most hemodialysis patients are asymptomatic and their hepatic diseases often spontaneously resolve, we feel that liver biopsy is rarely helpful because of its nonspecificity. We do not routinely perform biopsies in these patients.

Because of the frequency of anicteric viral hepatitis in dialysis patients and because of the difficulty in appreciating the early symptoms of hepatitis—symptoms that closely mimic those of uremia or the side effects of hemodialysis—doctors in many dialysis units routinely screen patients with liver function tests and determinations of Australia (Au) antigen [50-52]. The Au antigen was initially detected by immunodiffusion, as described by Blumberg and Prince [53,54], and later by counterimmunoelectrophoresis. This antigen was shown to be present in a high percentage of people from tropical populations, patients with Down's syndrome, Leukemia, and, later, hepatitis. Subsequently, many patients in hemodialysis units were found to have this antigen and it was concluded this represented the presence of hepatitis. A recently developed radioimmunoassay for detection of Australia antigen is extremely sensitive and detects the Au antigen and antibody 1 to 2 percent and 10 to 21 percent, respectively, more often than the counterimmunoelectrophoretic method [55]. Some reports have described symptoms of hepatitis milder in uremic than nonuremic patients and also a high incidence of chronic antigenemia in dialysis populations [50,56,57]. We had a large hepatitis epidemic [58] in which the symptoms in dialysis patients resembled those in the staff. Continued sporadic cases occur, but chronic antigenemia has been found in less than 2 percent, even when patients are screened by radioimmunoassay. We have been unable to correlate the presence of the antigen with other evidence of hepatitis, either in the patient or other contacts in the dialysis unit, and the significance or relevance of this sensitive test in uremic patients in hemodialysis units remains to be determined. In the meantime, such patients should be handled as potentially infectious.

To avoid introducing hepatitis into hemodialysis units, it is advisable to screen all incoming patients and new employees with liver enzyme tests and determination of Australia antigen. We feel that patients with positive Australia antigens who are otherwise well and are suitable transplant or dialysis candidates should be admitted to the program. Employees with positive Australia antigens may be excellent potential dialyzers after conversion of positive antigenemia, because of their resulting immunity.

After using both the SGOT and Australia antigen to screen a large dialysis population at monthly intervals over a 3-year period, we found Australia antigen screening *alone* to yield very few unsuspected cases. We currently screen with SGOT's or SGPT's and obtain tests for Australia antigen only in those patients with symptoms or elevated enzymes to help in the differential diagnosis, or routinely every three months. Since Australia antigen positivity occurs early and usually before elevation of SGOT, we may miss some cases of "hepatitis" in which there is a brief elevation of the antigen titer. This may not be significant, as pointed out above, since the brief period of positive antigenemia seems to have little effect on either the patient or the subsequent incidence of viral hepatitis in patients or staff. Asymptomatic patients with elevated liver enzymes but with negative Australia antigen are observed without further precautions. Any patient whose clinical picture strongly suggests hepatitis must be treated as infectious, even in the absence of a positive Australia antigen.

Most dialysis centers now transfuse patients only when symptoms of anemia are severe. Continued efforts to reduce the number of blood transfusions are important if hepatitis is to be controlled. Tullis et al [59] demonstrated a decreased incidence of hepatitis using previously frozen red blood cells, and using frozen blood when transfusions are necessary should help in reducing the incidence of hepatitis. Protection is not complete, however, as we have identified Australia antigen positivity in several patients who either never received blood transfusions or who received *only* frozen red blood cells.

Nurses and technicians dialyzing more than 1 patient should wear gloves while handling blood products, lines, or other blood-contaminated sources and should change gloves from patient to patient. Aprons and other protective clothing should be worn and discarded after the dialysis, and contaminated clothing should be changed after the nurse or technician leaves the dialysis unit. Patients and nurses should have separate toilet and washing facilities. The walls, floors, and ancillary equipment should be cleaned regularly and throughly, and blood-exposed dialysis equipment should be cleaned with either gluteraldehyde or 2 percent formaldehyde at least at weekly intervals. Frequent and repeated education of the patients and nursing staff in hygiene and aseptic techniques is necessary. Patients who already have developed hepatitis or who are admitted to the dialysis unit with Australia antigen might best be isolated to particular dialysis machines designated for use in hepatitis patients. The nursing and dialyzing staff should use special care in the dialysis of such patients, although all patients in a dialysis unit should be treated as if they were infectious. Patients with hepatitis need not be removed from the dialysis unit but can be isolated within the unit by means of careful nursing procedures.

Although hyperimmune globulin is of questionable value in type B or long-incubation, Australia antigen-positive hepatitis [60-62], it may help reduce the severity in contacts of type A, short-incubation hepatitis [63,64]. When an operator's skin is broken or he becomes considerably contaminated with blood from suspected hepatitis patients, he should be given hyperimmune gammaglobulin, since the differential of type A and type B hepatitis is difficult to determine.

The incidence of hepatitis in home dialysis patients should be less than in center patients; however, we have known 3 dialyzing spouses to develop hepatitis. Aseptic techniques cannot be overemphasized in the home training program. We do not feel that it is justifiable to place a patient with known hepatitis in the home, thereby placing the burden squarely on the family.

Briggs et al [58] reported the effect of hepatitis in patients before and after transplantation and concluded that the severity of hepatitis in the transplanted patient is not as bad as had been previously suggested [65]. We feel that patients who have had hepatitis are suitable candidates for transplantation, even though chronic positive antigenemia has been found to be much greater in these immunosuppressed patients. The morbidity from chronic positive antigenemia in transplant patients appears inconsequential. It should be pointed out, however, that there has been no long-term follow-up of these patients and subsequent complications such as chronic active hepatitis and cirrhosis have not had time to develop. In summary, hepatitis remains one of the major complications of chronic hemodialysis; however, if properly managed, it may not be as severe as previously anticipated. With the advent of more specific screening methods, possibilities of immunization [66], and continued epidemiologic surveillance, the problem of hepatitis will hopefully become inconsequential.

REFERENCES

1. Jaffe, R.H., Laing, N.R.: Changes of the digestive tract in uremia. A pathologic anatomic study. Ann Intern Med 53:851, 1934.
2. Bailey, G.L., Griffiths, H.J., Lock, J.P., et al: Gastrointestinal abnormalities in uremia (abstract), Am Soc Nephrology 5th Annual Meeting, Nov. 1971, p 5.
3. Comty, C.M., Baillod, R.A., Shaldon, S.: Two and one-half years experience with a nurse-patient operated chronic dialysis unit. Proc Europ Dial Transpl Assoc 2:88, 1965.
4. Schupak E., Merrill, J.P.: Experience with long-term intermittent hemodialysis. Ann Intern Med 62:509, 1965.
5. Pendras, J.P., Erickson, R.U.: Hemodialysis: A successful therapy for chronic uremia. Ann Intern Med 64:293, 1966.
6. Hampers, C.L., Schupak, E.: Gastrointestinal Function, in Long-Term Hemodialysis, The Management of the Patient with Chronic Renal Failure. New York, Grune & Stratton, 1967, p 135.
7. Boner, G., Berry, E.M.: Gastrointestinal hemorrhage complicating chronic hemodialysis. Isr J Med Sci 4:66, 1968.
8. Moynihan, B.G.A.: Uremic ulcer of the duodenum, in Peptic Ulcer. ed 2, Philadelphia, W.B. Saunders Co., 1912, pp 44-67.
9. Wiener, S.N., Vertes, V., Shapiro, H.: The upper gastrointestinal tract in patients undergoing chronic dialysis. Radiology 92:110, 1969.
10. Meschan, I.: Roentgen signs in clinical practice. Philadelphia, W.B. Saunders Co., vol 2, 1966, p 1520.
11. Hennessy, W.J., Siemsen, A.W.: Autonomic neuropathy in chronic renal failure. Clin Res 16:385, 1968.
12. Goldenberger, S., Thompson, A., Guha, A.: Autonomic nervous dysfunction in chronic renal failure. Clin Res 19:531, 1971.
13. Lazarus, J.M., Hampers, C.L., Lowrie, E.G., et al: Baroreceptor activity in normotensive and hypertensive uremic patients. Circulation (in press).

14. Van den Bogaert, P., Pennoit, H., Elewaut, A., et al: Uremic gastritis. A study of twenty uremic patients with terminal renal insufficiency. Tijdschr Gastroenterol 15:125, 1972.

15. King, A.Y., Schneider, H.J., King, L.R.: The roentgen appearance of the small bowel during long-term hemodialysis for chronic renal disease. Radiology 99:331, 1971.

16. Blainey, J.D., Northam, B.E.: Amylase excretion by the human kidney. Clin Sci 32:377, 1967.

17. Bartos, V., Melichar, J., Erben, J.: The function of the exocrine pancreas in chronic renal failure. Digestion 3:33, 1970.

18. Lieber, C.S., Lefevre, A.: Ammonia as a source of gastric hypoacidity in patients with uremia. J Clin Invest 38:1271, 1959.

19. Mossberg, S.M., Thayer, W.B., Spiro, H.M.: Azotemia and gastric acidity: The effect of intravenous urea on gastric acid and gastric ammonia production in man. J Lab Clin Med 61:469, 1963.

20. Goldstein, H., Murphy, D., Sokol, A., et al: Gastric and acid secretion in patients undergoing chronic dialysis. Arch Intern Med 120:645, 1967.

21. Gingell, J.C., Burns, G.P., Chishold, G.D.: Gastric acid secretion in chronic uremia and after renal transplantation. Br Med J 4:424, 1968.

22. Hampers, C.L., Schupak, E.: Gastrointestinal Function, in Long-Term Hemodialysis. New York, Grune & Stratton, 1967, p 137.

23. Ventkateswaren, P.S., Jeffers, A., Hocken, A.G.: Gastric acid secretion in chronic renal failure. Br Med J 4:22, 1972.

24. Fillastre, J.P., Blaise, P., Ardaillou, R., et al: Secretion gastrique des uremics. Rev Eur Etud Clin Biol 10:188, 1965.

25. Murphy, D.L., Goldstein, H., Boyle, J.B., et al: Hypercalcemia and gastric secretion in man. J Appl Physiol 21:1607, 1966.

26. Ward, J.T., Adesola, A.O., Welbourn, R.B.: The parathyroids, calcium and gastric secretion in man and the dog. Gut 5:173, 1964.

27. Barreras, R.F., Donaldson, R.M.: Role of calcium in gastric hypersecretion, parathyroid adenoma and peptic ulcer. N Engl J Med 276: 1122, 1967.

28. Durkin, M.G., Essig, L.J., Nolph, K.D.: Gastrin removal during peritoneal dialysis. Clin Res 19:657, 1971.

29. Maxwell, J.G., Moore, J.L., Dixon, J., et al: Gastrin levels in anephric patients. Surg Forum 22:305, 1971.

30. Korman, M.G., Laver, M.D., Hansky, J.: Hypergastrinaemia in chronic renal failure. Br Med J 1:209, 1972.

31. Reeder, D.D., Thompson, J.D.: Effect of hemodialysis on serum gastrin levels in uremic patients. (abstract) Gastroenterology 60:795, 1971.

32. Lewicki, A.M., Saito, S., Merrill, J.P.: Gastrointestinal bleeding in the renal transplant patient. Radiology 102:533, 1972.

33. Penn, I., Groth, C.F., Brettschneider, L., et al: Surgically correctable intra-abdominal complications before and after renal hemotransplantation. Ann Surg 168:865, 1968.

34. Gordon, E.M., Johnson, A.G., Williams, G.: Gastric assessment of prospective renal-transplant patients. Lancet 2:226, 1972.

35. Hadjiyannakis, E.J., Evans, D.B., Smellie, W.A.B., et al: Gastrointestinal complications after renal transplantation. Lancet 2:781, 1971.
36. Coleman, M.J., Lord, R.S.A., Hayes, J., et al: Renal transplantation in South Australia. Med J Aust 1:546, 1972.
37. Cooke, A.R.: Corticosteroids and peptic ulcer: Is there a relationship? Am J Dig Dis 12:232, 1967.
38. Berlyne, G.M., Ben-Ari, J., Pest, D., et al: Hyperaluminaemia from aluminum resins in renal failure. Lancet 2:494, 1970.
39. Pastor, B., Resnick, M.E., Rodman, T.: Serious hemorrhagic complication of anticoagulant therapy. JAMA 180:747, 1962.
40. Goldfarb, W.B.: Coumarin-induced intestinal obstruction. Ann Surg 161:27, 1965.
41. Crisler, C., Stafford, E.S., Zuidema, G.D.: Intestinal obstruction in patients receiving anticoagulants. Surg Clin North Am 50:1009, 1970.
42. DeSanto, N.G., Capodicasa, G., Perna, N., et al: Haematoma of rectus abdominis associated with dialysis. Br Med J 3:281, 1972.
43. Hampers, C.L., Schupak, E.: Gastrointestinal Function, in Long-Term Hemodialysis. New York, Grune & Stratton, 1967.
44. Zerafos, N., Duffy, B., Chrysant, S., et al: Dialysis ascites: A new syndrome? (abstract), Fifth Intern Congress of Nephrology, Mexico City, Mexico, Abstract #34, 1972.
45. Mahony, J., Pinggera, W., Holmes, J., et al: Ascites during maintenance hemodialysis. (abstract), Fifth Intern Congress of Nephrology, Mexico City, Mexico, Abstract #64, 1972.
46. Versaci, A.A., Soriano, R.U., Mao, R.L., et al: Serum enzymes in chronic hemodialysis. Chicago Med Sch Quart 27:222, 1968.
47. Bailey, G.L., Katz, A.I., Hampers, C.L., et al: Alterations in serum enzymes in chronic renal failure. JAMA 213:2263, 1970.
48. Sherlock, S.: Post-operative jaundice, in *Diseases of the Livary and Biliary System,* ed 4. Oxford, Blackwell, 1965, p 471.
49. Bergman, L.A., Thomas, W., Reddy, C.R., et al: Non-viral hepatitis in patients maintained by long term dialysis. Arch Intern Med 130:96, 1972.
50. Turner, G.C., White, G.B.B.: S.H. antigen in haemodialysis-associated hepatitis. Lancet 2:121, 1969.
51. Knight, A.H., Fox, R.A., Baillod, R.A., et al: Hepatitis-associated antigen and antibody in haemodialysis patients and staff. Br Med J 3:603, 1970.
52. Hepatitis and the treatment of chronic renal failure. Report of the Advisory Group, Dept of Health & Social Security, Scottish Home & Health Dept., Welsh Office, 1970-1972.
53. Blumberg, B.S., Alter, H.J., Visnich, S.: A "new" antigen in leukemia sera. JAMA 191:101, 1965.
54. Prince, A.M.: Relation of australia and SH antigens. Lancet 2:462, 1968.
55. Hacker, E.J., Aach, R.D.: Detection of hepatitis-associated antigen and anti-HAA. Comparison of radioimmunoassay and counterimmunoelectrophoresis. JAMA 223:414, 1973.

56. London, W.T., Difiglia, M., Sutnick, A.I., et al: An epidemic of hepatitis in a chronic-hemodialysis unit. N Engl J Med 281:571, 1968.
57. Nordenfeldt, E., Kjellen, L.: Presence and persistence of australia antigen in a Swedish hepatitis series. Acta Pathol Microbiol Scand 77:489, 1969.
58. Briggs, W.A., Lazarus, J.M., Birtch, A.G., et al: Considerations and consequences of hepatitis affecting hemodialysis and transplant patients. Arch Intern Med(in press).
59. Tullis, J.L., Hinman, J., Sproul, M.T., et al: Incidence of post-transfusion hepatitis in previously frozen blood. JAMA 214:719, 1970.
60. Hepatitis surveillance. Center for Disease Contr., Ref. #33, U.S. Dept. Health, Education and Welfare, Public Health Service, Jan. 1, 1971.
61. Grady, G.F., Bennett, A.J.E.: Cooperative study: prevention of post-transfusion hepatitis by gamma globulin. JAMA 214:140, 1970.
62. Ginsberg, A.L., Conrad, M.E., Bancroft, W.H., et al: Prevention of endemic HAA-positive hepatitis with gamma globulin. N Engl J Med 286:562, 1972.
63. Stokes, J., Neefe, J.R.: The prevention and attenuation of infectious hepatitis by gamma globulin. JAMA 127:144, 1945.
64. Advisory Committee on Immunizing Practices. U.S. Public Health Service Meeting, June, 1968: Immune serum globulin for prevention of viral hepatitis. Ann Intern Med 69:1009, 1968.
65. Moore, T.C., Hume, A.M.: The period and nature of hazard in clinical renal transplantation. Ann Surg 170:1, 1969.
66. Krugman, S., Giles, J.P., Hammond, J.: Viral hepatitis, type B (MS-2 strain) studies on active immunization. JAMA 217:41, 1971.

8
The Neurological System

Nuerological abnormalities as a consequence of uremia are well known. However, prior to chronic dialysis they had been thought of primarily as involving the central nervous system and included those signs leading up to uremic coma—lethargy, somnolence, irritability, restlessness, fasciculations, asterixis, confusion, and convulsions. Peripheral nerve dysfunction, a more recently recognized complication of chronic renal failure, has received increasing attention since the advent of dialysis [1,2]. Neurologic deficits resulting from chronic renal failure may be present prior to initiation of dialysis, may appear shortly after dialysis has begun, or may first appear later, after a patient has already been stabilized.

Excellent reviews of the neurologic disorders in renal failure have been published by Tyler [3,4]. Mild defects of mentation are common, sometimes even with only mild uremia, and these initially mild symptoms may progress with increasing uremia as indicated above to disorientation, delusions, and even frank psychosis, which, when associated with dialysis, may take many days to resolve. The form that the neurological abnormality takes frequently depends on the patient's underlying personality structure. Any or all of the neurological disorders in renal failure may be aggravated or even instigated by rapid dialysis.

CENTRAL NERVOUS SYSTEM DYSFUNCTION

Central nervous system dysfunction may be noted in patients with severe renal failure prior to, during, or immediately following hemodialysis. These disturbances, more common in the early phase of dialytic treatment and in patients with acute renal failure, may also occur in individuals who have had many uneventful dialyses previously. Headache, nausea, vomiting, restlessness, agitation, rising blood pressure, confusion and even frank grand mal seizures may be seen. These manifestations are more likely to appear when the patient has undergone very efficient dialysis; they are more common in the elderly and in the sick. However, they may occur at any time—even after the most gentle dialysis. The syndrome of cerebral dysfunction occurring with or after dialysis has come to be known as the "disequilibrium syndrome" [5,6]. The cause of this dysfunction is not completely clear, but most experimental work suggests that a rapid lowering of the serum urea plays a major role [7-9]. With an acute reduction in the level of blood urea, insufficient time is allowed for an equal reduction of urea in the cerebrospinal fluid. Because of the slow transport of urea across the "blood-brain barrier," an osmotic gradient is produced in which water moves from the blood and extracellular fluid into the central nervous system. Measurements of blood and spinal fluid urea nitrogen after dialysis indicate that the urea concentration may be significantly higher in the spinal fluid than in the blood [6,8]. A "reverse urea effect" is produced and water moves down the osmotic gradient into the central nervous system. Experiments in animals substantiate this theory by demonstrating an increase in cerebrospinal fluid pressure during rapid hemodialysis [10]. Other animal studies comparing dialysis with a high urea concentrate in the dialysate with dialysis fluid without urea demonstrated increased cisternal pressure only when dialysis was performed against a urea-free bath [11]. Scribner has noted tensing of a brain flap in a neurosurgical patient undergoing hemodialysis [12]. This evidence and experiments performed by others indicates that an increase in cerebrospinal fluid pressure plays an important role in the disequilibrium syndrome. The cause of the increased pressure, however, is still in doubt.

Electroencephalographic disturbances usually parallel the clinical disorder (see Fig. 1). Kennedy and colleagues found a marked deterioration in EEG tracings obtained during and immediately following dialysis [5]. Although they did not measure cerebrospinal fluid changes, they were able to protect against a deteriorating EEG by adding an osmotically active substance to the dialysis fluid or by intravenously infusing

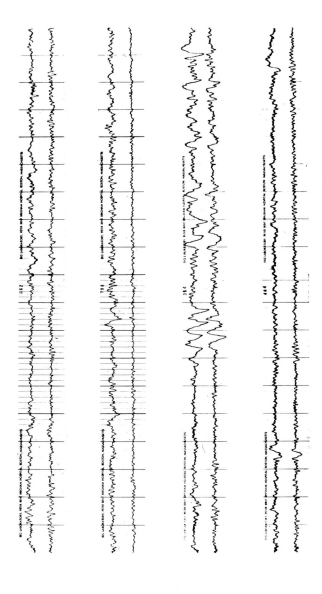

Fig. 1. EEG (right-sided bipolar leads taken from frontal and frontal-cerebral areas) on 4 consecutive days in patient with moderate uremia. On third day without any detectable change in clinical or chemical status, EEG deteriorated. Note slowing and rare paroxysmal discharge. The tracing subsequently spontaneously improved.

157

fructose into the patient during dialysis [14]. In a recent study in which uremic animals underwent rapid hemodialysis, it was shown by means of brain biopsy that these animals developed cerebral swelling in both cortex and white matter [9]. The authors concluded that this swelling was due to osmotic forces associated with rapid removal of the urea from the extracellular fluid.

The available evidence that urea is a significant factor in the disequilibrium syndrome is compelling. However, not all investigators agree that this is the only factor [15,16]. During rapid hemodialysis changes—such as acid-base changes, rapid shifts of ions, or cardiovascular alterations—in various areas affect body homeostasis, and any or all of these can affect central nervous system function. In our most recent experience [17] there has been no consistent correlation between an increase in cerebrospinal fluid pressure or osmolality and clinical or electroencephalographic changes of the "disequilibrium syndrome." Both would have been expected if the syndrome were due simply to a "reverse urea effect."

Robin and colleagues [18] have measured acid-base parameters during artifically induced respiratory acidosis, respiratory alkalosis, metabolic acidosis, and metabolic alkalosis. They showed that in respiratory acidosis and alkalosis, the pH of the blood and cerebrospinal fluid fluctuate together in accordance with changes in pCO_2, but during metabolic acidosis and alkalosis, the change in bicarbonate is not immediately reflected in the cerebrospinal fluid. These findings can be explained by postulating a relative impermeability of the blood-brain barrier to bicarbonate with free diffusion of carbon dioxide. The changes found after hemodialysis are consistent with such an assumption. The bicarbonate level in the cerebrospinal fluid is slightly greater than that of the blood before dialysis. Bicarbonate concentration in spinal fluid remains relatively constant during dialysis in spite of an increase in blood bicarbonate. Therefore, following dialysis most patients demonstrate a relative alkalosis in the blood with little change in spinal fluid pH. Factors influencing cerebrospinal fluid pH have been summarized by Posner, Swanson, and Plum [19]. The magnitude of the acid-base change in the blood and spinal fluid resulting from dialysis can vary considerably and must be considered at least a potential contributor to the disequilibrium syndrome.

Arieff and Massry [20] studied the dialysis disequilibrium syndrome. Various measurements were performed and the experiments were done in normal dogs and uremic dogs treated with slow and rapid hemodialysis. Their data suggest that rapid hemodialysis in uremic animals is associated with the accumulation of "idiogenic osmoles" in the brain, which results in an osmotic gradient between brain and plasma. This in turn causes cerebral edema, increased intracranial pressure, and seizures. Although this study does not elucidate the nature of idiogenic osmoles, it does suggest that there may be an increased formation of organic acid radicals in the brain which is reflected by the fall in CSF pH and is observed after rapid hemodialysis. It further suggests that there may be intercellular changes such as binding of cations $(K+$ or $Na+)$ as a result of changes in intercellular pH. Further data are needed to clarify these findings, but they are interesting from a pathophysiologic standpoint.

The EEG changes of chronic renal failure are not specific and have been reported by several authors [21,22]. These changes are characterized by disturbances of cortical background rhythm with replacement or intermingling of the normal alpha waves by irregular activity of slower rhythm. In addition, some patients show paroxysms of synchronous slow waves at 4 to 6 per second or less. During dialysis the EEG will be noted to deteriorate as manifested by a further decrease in alpha activity and increase in theta- and delta-range waves. The record taken 24 hours postdialysis generally shows considerable improvement over the postdialysis tracing.

It should be emphasized at this point that with improvement in dialysis technique—including increased efficiency, and more frequent dialysis—EEG changes during and subsequent to dialysis are much less common.

Kennedy and co-workers have demonstrated the value of glucose in preventing dialysis-induced EEG changes [5,14]. This protection may be effected as a result of the increase of osmolality of the bath and a resultant decrease in cerebrospinal fluid pressure. However, it does appear that in patients with chronic renal failure, cerebral glucose consumption is reduced [23] (exemplified by decreased oxygen utilization without consistent changes in cerebral blood flow), and this may be related to an interference with cerebral carbohydrate metabolism. Increasing the concentration of cerebrospinal fluid glucose—as is accomplished by performing dialysis against a high dialysate-glucose concentration—may beneficially affect cerebral metabolism separate from its osmotic activity, and this in turn might be reflected by a more normal EEG.

Treatment of the disequilibrium syndrome should be aimed at prevention. This is frequently best accomplished by a slow, gradual readjustment of body chemistry toward normalcy, which may be achieved with either peritoneal or hemodialysis, although both should be brief and relatively inefficient. Nevertheless, even with peritoneal dialysis, disequilibrium may occur. When hemodialysis is employed as the initial treatment modality, dialysis should be short and at frequent intervals with low blood flows. It would also seem prudent to add glucose to the dialysis bath. Despite this, disequilibrium may still take place and appropriate preventive measures are indicated. Ideally, overtly uremic patients should receive diphenylhydantoin (Dilantin) at least 24 hours prior to dialysis. However, this is not always possible and sometimes Dilantin cannot be administered until just before dialysis. In such circumstances we have not hesitated to give from 500 to 1,000 mg intramuscularly as a single dose. Phenobarbitol or diazepam (Valium) may also be used as premedicants. In the event of frank seizures, intravenous Dilantin may be of value, although Valium or a rapid-acting barbiturate, such as amobarbital, administered intravenously seems to be the drug of choice.

If early signs of disequilibrium appear, it is wise to terminate dialysis and administer drugs as described above. One may also alleviate symptomatology at times with the administration of hypertonic glucose. Sometimes manifestations of disequilibrium persist for up to 24 hours or, rarely, 48 hours postdialysis. Aside from those measures designed to minimize the likelihood of convulsions, there is nothing specific to be done other than provide supportive therapy.

A common physical finding in the uremic patient and in the patient with the dialysis disequilibrium syndrome is asterixis, characterized by a flop of the dorsiflexed hand. Tyler [3] suggests that the defect is a periodic inhibition of muscular contraction (dorsiflexion) which probably originates above the spinal motor neuron pool and affects a single limb. In patients with mild to moderate renal failure, muscular cramps occur frequently. Occasionally, these may be due to sodium depletion but frequently there is no apparent correlation with any abnormality in serum electrolytes. The subject of muscle cramps is discussed further in Chapter 10. Muscular hyperirritability in the form of fasciculations is common. True tetanic phenomena are not common and are rarely related to hypocalcemia; they reflect the more generalized metabolic disturbances of the central nervous system. One exception to this may be the production of tetany by the rapid infusion of bicarbonate in an acidotic patient with hypocalcemia. The resultant acute alkalosis may result in true hypocalcemia tetany.

PERIPHERAL NEUROPATHY

With the increasing applicability and success of chronic hemodialysis, there has been an increasing awareness and a greater incidence of peripheral nerve dysfunction. The neurologic involvement, when it occurs, is typically symmetrical, beginning distally at the toes and spreading up the leg [24]. Upper extremity involvement, seen only in the face of severe lower extremity involvement, develops insidiously and in the majority of patients is manifested solely by reduction in nerve conduction. Only in its severest stages is clinical symptomatology present. Then the neuropathy may be characterized by pain and paresthesias of the lower extremities, a marked sensitivity to touch, and a "burning" feeling. Although sensory manifestations of the disease may initially indicate the patient's involvement, there may be a significant motor component as well. In some cases the motor component is the most prominent finding, and the patient's first knowledge of his involvement is difficulty with walking.   Rarely do the lower extremities become totally paralyzed.

One of the earliest signs of peripheral neuropathy may be the restless leg syndrome [25] in which the patient feels uncomfortable when at rest, so he thrashes about in an effort to find relief. Relief may be obtained by moving the leg or walking. For some reason this syndrome is more common during dialysis, and in a few instances we have had to discontinue dialysis because of severe patient discomfort. We have not observed the restless leg syndrome in the absence of diminished nerve conduction velocity.

The burning feet syndrome, perhaps another manifestation of peripheral neuropathy, is characterized by a painful, burning paresthesia of the feet, generally bilaterally, and generally severely curtailing ambulation. Patients are acutely uncomfortable and suffer harsh pain from the slightest stimulation.

The pathologic abnormalities found in the peripheal nerves cannot be distinguished from those which occur in diabetes mellitus or chronic alcoholism [26]. There is generally extensive demyelination, most marked distally. Nerve fiber sheaths may be swollen and, in places, fragmented. Usually there are large numbers of fat-laden macrophages and a conspicuous absence of infiltration of inflammatory cells.

The etiology of peripheral neuropathy is as poorly understood, as is the etiology of uremia itself. Although it was originally postulated that neuropathy was in some way attributable to hemodialysis and vitamin depletion might be responsible [27], it now appears quite evident that the neuropathy results from the further evolution of uremia and is a consequence of the progression of disease. That it is unrelated to the level of urea nitrogen has been amply demonstrated by Lonergan, Semar, and Lange [28]. By imposing severe dietary restrictions on patients and offering hemodialysis on an infrequent basis, they were able to maintain people with relatively low levels of urea nitrogen, yet observe significant advancement of peripheral neuropathy. Similar observations have been made by others in patients denied dialysis and given various protein-restricted diets [29].

What role, if any, nutritional factors play in peripheral neuropathy is likewise unknown. Although vitamins have been found to be decreased in patients maintained by dialysis—and indeed, water-soluble vitamins are removed by dialysis [27]—the peripheral neuropathy present in dialysis patients does not respond to even massive vitamin replacement [30].

Peripheral neuropathy has been adjudged by some to be a manifestation and a consequence of inadequate dialysis. This is undoubtedly true in some instances. However, a significant percentage of patients referred to us for maintenance dialysis therapy already have demonstrable neuropathy, at least as measured by nerve conduction times. The incidence and severity of neuropathy usually depend upon the timeliness of the referral for dialysis. The longer the patient remains uremic, the more likely and the more severe the neuropathy will be.

Among other indicators of the need for dialysis, we rely upon abnormal nerve conduction times, even in the absence of clinical neuropathy. In patients followed in our renal clinics prior to the initiation of dialysis, sequential nerve conduction studies are obtained as one means of determining the appropriate time to initiate treatment (Figs. 2 and 3). We have not hesitated to initiate dialysis when patients have been asymptomatic but had abnormal nerve conduction times. The results achieved in these patients over a period of several years have been most gratifying and conclusively support our judgment in providing early treatment. Furthermore, patients started on dialysis prior to the development of signs and symptoms of uremia have unquestionably had a lower incidence of morbidity and mortality than patients in whom treatment was delayed.

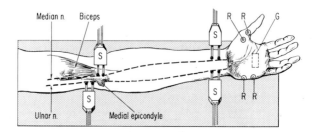

Fig. 2. Drawing of arm indicating relation of median and ulnar nerves and positions of simulating electrodes *(S)* at wrist and elbow. Recording electrodes *(R)* are shown in position for recording responses to median and ulnar nerve stimulation. Ground electrode *(G)* is placed on back of hand.

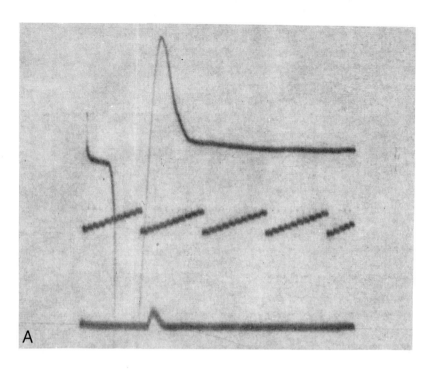

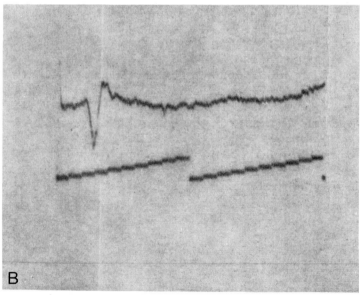

Fig. 3. (A). Muscle action potential elicited by stimulating median nerve at wrist. (B). Sensory nerve action potential elicited by stimulating ulnar nerve at wrist.

Although there is some general relationship of neuropathy to renal function as measured by either serum creatinine or creatinine clearance, it is at best a poor one. Recognizing the variability and fluctuation observed in individual nerve conduction studies [31], we nevertheless have found them useful in assessing both the progression of uremia prior to dialysis and the subsequent adequacy of dialysis. Sequential deterioration in nerve conduction studies in patients already undergoing dialysis has indicated that dialysis was inadequate and we have responded with an increase in dialysis time or frequency or both. We now recognize that the amount of dialysis required may vary in a given patient with a change in clinical status. With an increase in metabolic rate or in the presence of severe illness with increased catabolism, dialysis requirements increase. In previously stable patients, we have observed progressive deterioration in nerve conduction time subsequent to the development of acute medical problems. We now adjust dialysis time upward on an acute basis to meet the anticipated increased need.

To properly use nerve conduction studies and derive meaningful information from them, sequential studies must be performed. It should also be noted that surgical procedures designed to obtain access to the blood supply may temporarily or permanently interfere with nerve conduction velocity.

Peripheral neuropathy in the predialysis or dialysis patient may be reversible if detected and treated sufficiently early. We have been able to demonstrate this with nerve conduction studies and have even observed reversal of foot drop. The key factor is early detection and vigorous treatment before irreversible changes take place.

When a sudden worsening in nerve conduction time is detected or when neuropathy suddenly appears, we significantly increase dialysis time. For example, when it has been indicated, we have dialyzed patients for from 50 to 100 percent longer with a similar increase in frequency. Our results have generally but not always been favorable. We have observed patients who have undergone twin-coil dialysis for 8 hours 4 or 5 times a week without improvement. We have also witnessed patients similarly treated whose clinical nerve conduction improved dramatically.

In a few instances, patients have undergone prolonged extra dialysis without any demonstrable improvement in nerve conduction time, but with a slow yet definite improvement of clinical symptomatology. Most noticeable in patients with burning and painful feet, this is usually attributable to improved muscle strength and reflects efforts toward physical rehabilitation. The importance of physical rehabilitation in the overall management of the dialysis patient cannot be overemphasized.

OTHER INVOLVEMENT

Although central and peripheral nervous system involvement in uremia are well accepted, autonomic nervous system function has been studied little. Some evidence indicates that barorceptor function is deranged in patients with renal failure [32-35] and that this may be related to uremia per se [34]. In studying dialyzed patients with and without significant hypertension and utilizing the pulse response to a controlled increase in blood pressure as an indication of autonomic nervous system function, we found an abnormal response in all cases [34]. Ordinarily, an increase in blood pressure results in a predicatable slowing of heart rate, and this "slope" can be shown to be deranged in patients maintained with the artificial kidney. It does not appear likely from our preliminary data that this deranged autonomic function will improve with intensification of dialysis, and its contribution to general well-being is unknown. Nevertheless, this type of derangement is an indication that patients maintained with dialysis are not totally well and may still suffer from low-level uremic problems. This point may be further substantiated by electroencephalographic studies performed by Kiley and co-workers [36,37], which demonstrated that the electroencephalogram in many patients maintained on *twice* weekly dialysis remained abnormal. Although the electroencephalogram improved with regular dialysis, the fact that it was not normal is of interest. Further studies performed on patients on *three* times a week dialysis show considerably improved EEG's. Whether all electroencephalographic changes disappear with *daily* dialysis is conjecture and these findings are cited as another example that some low level of uremia probably persists despite what is currently considered "adequate" dialysis.

Ginn and associates [38] have now begun to study neurobehavioral and clinical responses to hemodialysis in an attempt to analyze and evaluate the results of certain dialysis schedules and determine an appropriate treatment. They were able to quatify, at least in part, several neuro-behavioral manifestations of uremia. In patients studied, neurophysiological and psychological abnormalities tended to vary *within* patients directly with time and inversely following dialysis and 2) *between* patients according to dialysis schedules. In patients with creatinine clearances below 2 ml/min, both within- and between-patient neurobehavioral test results were worse during twice weekly than during thrice weekly dialysis. Conventional laboratory measurements including urea and creatinine and bicarbonate concentrations as well as erythrocyte transketolase activity levels did not correlate with the neurobehavioral measurements. Moreover, intercorrelations of the several variables with the clinical observations raised serious questions concerning reliability of conventional bedside clinical assessment of the adequacy of dialysis and control of uremia. This strengthens the observation known by most physicians caring for dialysis patients that the overall clinical condition is far more important than any specific measurable laboratory test. All of these factors must be considered together in an individual patient.

REFERENCES

1. Marin, O.S.M., Tyler, H.R.: Hereditary interstitial nephritis associated with polyneuropathy. Neurology (Minneap) 11:999, 1961.
2. Tenckhoff, H.A., Boen, F.S.T., Jebsen, R.M., et al: Polyneuropathy in chronic renal insufficiency. JAMA 191:1121, 1965.
3. Tyler, H.R.: Neurological complications of acute and chronic renal failure. *Treatment of Renal Failure,* ed 2. New York, Grune & Stratton, 1965, p 315.
4. Tyler, H.R.: Neurological disorders in renal failure. Am J Med 44:734, 1968.
5. Kennedy, A.C., Linton, A.L., Luke, R.G., et al: Electroencephalographic changes during hemodialysis. Lancet 1:408, 1963.
6. Rosen, S.M., O'Connor, K., Shaldon, S.: Haemodialysis disequilibrium. Br Med J 2:672, 1964.
7. Peterson, H., Swanson, A.G.: Acute encephalopathy occurring during renal hemodialysis—the reverse urea effect. Arch Intern Med 113:877, 1964.
8. Kennedy, A.C., Linton, A.L., Eaton, J.C.: Urea levels in cerebrospinal fluid after hemodialysis. Lancet 1:410, 1962.
9. Dosseter, J.B., Oh, J.H., Dayes, L., et al: Brain urea and water changes with rapid hemodialysis of uremic dogs. Trans Am Soc Artif Intern Organs 10:323, 1964.
10. Sitprija, V., Holmes, J.H.: Preliminary observations on the change in intracranial pressure and intraocular pressure during hemodialysis. Trans Am Soc Artif Intern Organs 8:300, 1962.
11. Gilliland, K.G., Hegstrom, R.M.: The effect of hemodialysis on cerebrospinal fluid pressure in uremic dogs. Trans Am Soc Artif Intern Organs 9:44, 1963.
12. Scribner, B.H.: Discussion. Trans Am Soc Artif Intern Organs 8:195, 1962.

13. Peterson, H., Swanson, A.G.: Acute encephalopathy occurring during hemodialysis. Arch Intern Med 113:877, 1964.
14. Kennedy, A.C., Linton, A.L., Renfrew, S., et al: The pathogenesis and prevention of cerebral dysfunction during dialysis. Lancet 6:790, 1964.
15. Brun, D.: Discussion. Trans Am Soc Artif Intern Organs 10:331, 1964.
16. Durr, F., Zysno, E., Nieth, H.:Influence of the extracorporeal hemodialysis on the electroencephalogram in acute and chronic renal failure. Klin Wochenschr 43:1140, 1965.
17. Hampers, C.L., Doak, P.B., Callaghan, M.N., et al: The electroencephalogram and spinal fluid during hemodialysis. Arch Intern Med 118: 340, 1966.
18. Robin, E.D., Whaley, R.D., Crump, et al: Acid-base relations between spinal fluid and arterial blood with special reference to control of ventilation. J Appl Physiol 13:385, 1958.
19. Posner, J.B., Swanson, A.G., Plum, F.: Acid-base balance in cerebrospinal fluid. Arch Neurol 12:479, 1965.
20. Arieff, A.I., Massry, S.G.: Investigations into the pathophysiology of the dialysis disequilibrium syndrome. In 6th Ann Contractor's Conf, Artif Kidney-Chronic Uremia Prog of NIAMD and Digestive Dis 1973, (Feb. 12-14), p. 35.
21. Klingler, M.: EEG observations in uremia. Electroencephalogr Clin Neurophysiol 6:519, 1954.
22. Jacob, J.C., Gloor, P., Elwan, O.H., et al: Electroencephalographic changes in chronic renal failure. Neurology (Minneap) 15:419, 1965.
23. Scheinberg, P.: Effects of uremia on cerebral blood flow and metabolism. Neurology 4:101, 1954.
24. Tyler, H.R., Gottlieb, A.: Peripheral neuropathy in uremia. Proc 8th Internat Cong of Neurol (Vienna) 1965.
25. Callaghan, N.: Restless legs syndrome in uremic neuropathy. Neurology (Minneap) 16:359, 1966.
26. Asbury, A.K., Victor, M., Adams, R.D.: Uremic polyneuropathy. Arch Neurol 8:413, 1963.
27. Lasker, N., Harvey, A., Baker, H.: Vitamin levels in hemodialysis and intermittent peritoneal dialysis. Trans Am Soc Artif Intern Organs 9: 51, 1963.
28. Lonergan, E.T., Semar, M., Lange, K.: A dialyzable toxic factor in uremia. Trans Am Soc Artif Intern Organs 16:269, 1970.
29. Sebsen, R.H., Tenckhoff, H., Honet, S.C.: Natural history of uremia polyneuropathy and effects of dialysis. N Engl J Med 277:327, 1967.
30. Pendras, J.P., Erickson, R.V.: Hemodialysis: A successful therapy for chronic uremia. Ann Intern Med 64:293, 1966.
31. Kominami, N., Tyler, H.R., Hampers, C.L., et al: Variations in motor nerve conduction velocity in normal and uremic patients. Arch Intern Med 128:235, 1971.
32. McCubbin, J.W., Green, J.H., Page, I.H.: Baroreceptor function in chronic renal hypertension. Circ Res 4:205, 1956.

33. Kazdi, P., Wennermark, J.R.: Baroreceptor and synthetic activity in experimental renal hypertension in the dog. Circulation 17:785, 1958.
34. Lazarus, J.M., Hampers, C.L., Lowrie, E.G., et al: Baroreceptor activity in normotensive and hypertensive uremic patients. Circulation (in press)
35. Soriano, G., Eisinger, R.P.: Abnormal response to the valsalva maneuver in patients on chronic hemodialysis. Nephron 9:251, 1972.
36. Kiley, J.E.: Electronic EEG frequency analysis for evaluation of uremia. In Proc 4th Ann Contractor's Conf. Artif Kidney-Chronic Uremia Prog of NIAMD, 1971, p. 129.
37. Kiley, J.E., Millora, A.B.: Electronic EEG frequency analysis for evaluation of uremia. In 6th Ann Contractor's Conference, Artif Kidney-Chronic Uremia Prog of NIAMD and Digestive Dis, 1973 (Feb. 12-14), p 36.
38. Ginn, H.E., Teschan, P.E., Freeman, M., et al: Neuro-behavorial and clinical responses to hemodialysis. In 6th Annual Contractor's Conf, Artif Kidney-Chronic Uremia Prog of NIAMD and Digestive Dis, 1973 (Feb. 12-14), p 32.

9
Metabolic Considerations

CARBOHYDRATE INTOLERANCE

Carbohydrate intolerance associated with chronic renal failure has been appreciated for almost 50 years [1,2]. In 1925, Lindner, Hiller, and Van Slyke [1] demonstrated an exaggerated and prolonged rise in blood sugar after the administration of oral glucose in patients with glomerulonephritis and severe renal insufficiency. Individuals with glomerulonephritis but without renal insufficiency and patients with chronic nephrosis, on the other hand, demonstrated no such abnormality. Zubrod and colleagues [3] pointed out an apparent paradox in this regard in the early 1950's by describing a diminution in the insulin requirements of diabetics with advancing renal failure. They summarized the course of 190 patients who came to autopsy at the Johns Hopkins Hospital. Patients with diabetic nephropathy were compared to diabetics without this complication. Those patients with renal disease required progressively less insulin as the renal disease progressed, while those without renal lesions required progressively more. Subsequent investigations into the physiology of glucose and insulin metabolism in patients with chronic renal failure has shed light on this apparent paradox.

It is clear that the abnormalities in carbohydrate metabolism which attend chronic renal failure are not due simply to diabetes mellitus. Between 65 and 100 percent of patients with untreated uremia exhibit some degree of carbohydrate intolerance, dependiing upon the sensitivity of test methods employed. As a general rule, the only consistently detectable derangement is an abnormal glucose tolerance test. Nevertheless, increased levels of fasting blood sugars may be observed, and mild fasting hyperinsulinemia is common. Ketonemia does not occur as a complication of uremic glucose intolerance. Furthermore, if microaneurysms are seen in the ocular fundus, genetic diabetes mellitus should be considered as the primary cause of any abnormality in carbohydrate metabolism.

While carbohydrate intolerance may be clinically the least troublesome of all uremic abnormalities, it may well provide key insights into the metabolic derangements of renal failure and their amelioration or correction by hemodialysis. There are no severe sequelae to the carbohydrate intolerance of renal failure except occasional hyperosmotic states that may complicate peritoneal or hemodialysis against high glucose concentrations. These relatively mild and infrequent consequences contrast to other more common and potentially serious manifestations of uremia (e.g., disorders of acid–base and electrolyte metabolism and complications of neuropathy, hyperparathyroidism, and fatigue that may attend anemia). Nonetheless, carbohydrates play a central role in energy metabolism and provide substrates for various synthetic processes. Carbohydrate intolerance is also an abnormality on which objective, precise data can be procured. Furthermore, it is improved or corrected by hemodialysis and, as such, may ultimately provide a useful tool in measuring the adequacy of therapy.

Abnormal carbohydrate tolerance is noted during both oral [4-11] and intravenous [6-18] glucose tolerance testing. Both tests tend to improve but may not be normalized by adequate hemodialysis [9,10,13,15-17]. Alfrey and associates [17] found that only one or two dialyses were required to improve various parameters of glucose utilization and insulin secretion during hemodialysis. They measured peak glucose and insulin concentrations during dialysis against dialysate containing 1500 mg/100 ml glucose and determined the rate at which plasma glucose declined at the conclusion of the treatment. By the second or third treatment, they found that blood glucose levels were lower, serum insulin levels were higher, and postdialysis declines in blood glucose were more rapid than they had been prior to therapy. Hampers and his colleagues [13], on the other hand, found that approximately 2 weeks of hemodialysis therapy were required to effect consistent improvement in an intravenous glucose tolerance test. Inasmuch as the former study involved sustained pancreatic stimulation and did not test the rate at which the pancreas responded to increments in blood sugar and the latter determined insulin responses to a pulse of glucose, the two are not, strictly speaking, comparable.

Table 1
Glucose K rates* in Normals and Uremic Individuals
Before and After Dialysis

Patient No.	Normal	Predialysis Uremic	Postdialysis Uremic
1	4.20	0.69	1.14
2	2.78	0.99†	1.11
3	2.10	0.60	1.77
4	2.37	0.51	1.27
5	2.51	0.89	2.27
6	1.33	1.29†	0.97
7	2.17	1.36	1.72
8	1.92	0.82	1.31
9	2.35	0.69	1.26
10	2.36	0.63†	0.75
11		0.83	2.02
12		1.07†	0.93
Mean	2.41	0.87	1.38
S.D.	0.74	0.27	0.47

*Exponential disappearance rate of glucose multiplied by -100.
†Differences in pre- and post-dialysis K rates not significant.
The difference between pre- and post-dialysis uremic patients is significant ($p < 0.01$), but postdialysis uremic patients are still significantly different from normal subjects ($p < 0.001$).

Table 1 illustrates the changes in intravenous glucose tolerance tests that may result from adequate dialysis and compares these tests to a matched normal control group [15]. All K rates were statistically determined and 8 of the 12 individuals showed an improvement in K rate with 2 weeks of adequate hemodialysis. However, while glucose utilization improves it does *not* reach levels attained by a group of matched normal individuals. Nonetheless, all but 2 in the postdialysis uremic group fall within the 95 percent confidence limits of "normal." This distinction between the group means and individuals within a group is important because any *post*dialysis uremic stands a reasonable probability of having a "normal" intravenous glucose tolerance test by the usual standards. As a group, however, dialysis patients do not seem to metabolize intravenous glucose with the same rapidity as do normal individuals.

Urea, acidosis, and starvation [6,9,13] do not appear to be the specific cause of the carbohydrate abnormality. Some investigators, however, have suggested that depletion of body potassium may be a cause [19]. The data for this conclusion are not strong, since hypokalemia has not been present when measured [9,13,15]. Indeed, determinations of intracellular and total body potassium fail to reveal low values in most dialysis patients [20,21].

In general, impaired glucose utilization may be explained by abnormal insulin secretion, impaired glucose utilization or a combination of both. It is generally thought that insulin secretion is normal in total amount, although perhaps inappropriately low for the prevailing degree of insulin sensitivity [13,15,16]. Hemodialysis tends to increase the magnitude of insulin release in response to a given glucose load [10,13,15-17]. Peak levels of insulin appear in the blood somewhat later in uremic individuals, implying that the *speed* of release is somewhat altered [13-15]. Hemodialysis improves this abnormality. Figure 1 illustrates the insulin levels attained in 12 patients with chronic renal failure before and after a period of hemodialysis and compares these with a closely matched, normal control group. Insulin levels tend to be higher after hemodialysis and are indeed even greater than normal. Prior to dialysis, serum insulin levels in uremic individuals are higher than normal only in the fasting state and again late in the test. This late elevation is likely due to slowed insulin degradation, as will be discussed below, rather than to continuing insulin secretion.

An index of pancreatic sensitivity to glucose may be obtained

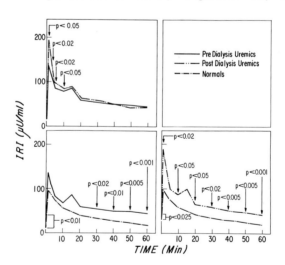

Fig. 1. Average immunoreactive insulin responses during an intravenous glucose tolerance test in 12 uremic patients before and after hemodialysis, and 10 matched normal controls. In uremic patients, immunoreactive insulin levels were higher after dialysis early in test and tended to be higher than those of normal subjects throughout test.

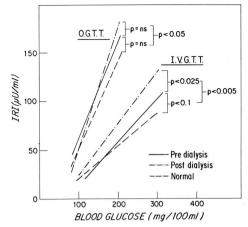

Fig. 2. Blood glucose-serum insulin relationships during oral and intravenous glucose tolerance tests in predialysis uremics, postdialysis uremics, and normal individuals. Serum insulin increment per given blood glucose increment was greater in uremics after dialysis than in normal subjects, and increment during intravenous glucose tolerance tests increased after dialysis in uremic individuals.

by determining the increment in serum insulin which accompanies a given increment in blood glucose. This determination is made by plotting blood glucose concentration against immunoreactive insulin levels. Figure 2 represents such a plot and compares uremic individuals before and after dialysis with normal subjects during both oral and intravenous glucose tolerance testing. In both instances, patients who have received adequate hemodialysis exhibit a greater increment in insulin for a given rise in blood glucose than do normal individuals. Patients with chronic renal failure who have not been dialyzed, on the other hand, are closer to normal individuals. A third finding, which suggests that insulin secretion is augmented by hemodialysis, is illustrated by Table 2. Again, 12 patients with chronic renal failure are compared to normal individuals. The initial 10-minute area and total area under the immunoreactive insulin versus time curves (as in Fig. 1) are compared for these groups. Hemodialysis significantly improves the amount of insulin secreted within the first 10 minutes. These curve areas are determined by the combined effects of insulin secretion and insulin degradation. Hence, increasing secretion or slowing degradation tends to increase the area. If one mathematically compensates for alterations in insulin degradation in an effort to estimate true secretion [16], these results are unchanged. However, the fraction of insulin secreted in

Table 2
Mean Urea Under IRI Versus Time Curves Above Fasting Levels*

Patient	10-Minute Area (μU min/ml)	60-Minute Area (μU min/ml)	$\dfrac{\textit{10-Minute area}}{\textit{60-Minute Area}} \times 100$
Predialysis uremic	615 ± 141†	2,196 ± 336	26.8 ± 3.3
Postdialysis uremic	852 ± 158†	2,789 ± 348‡	29.7 ± 2.9
Normal	619 ± 115	1,714 ± 267‡	36.8 ± 5.5

*Mean ± SEM

†Difference between means is significant (p < 0.001).

‡Difference between means is significant (p < 0.005).

the first 10 minutes (10-minute area per 60-minute area × 100) *is* changed. In predialysis patients, 36.2 percent of the area now resides in the first 10 minutes, while a similar value for dialyzed patients is 40.2 percent (p < 0.05).

This fraction of "early released" insulin may be an important correlate of glucose utilization [22]. If simple curve area alone is used, a correlation is observed in normals but not in patients with chronic renal failure. If alterations in insulin degradation are compensated by previously described methods [16] (in order to estimate true insulin secretion), a correlation between the fraction of insulin secreted in the first 10 minutes and K rate emerges for patients who have been dialyzed but not for those who have not, as shown in figure 3. In essence, this maneuver removes one more complicating variable—insulin degradation rate.

Rubenstein [23] and others have demonstrated that the kidneys play an important role in the metabolism of circulating insulin. The renal clearance of insulin in man is approximately 200 ml/min and the concentration of insulin renal venous blood is 30 to 40 percent lower than in arterial blood. O'Brien and Sharpe [24] have estimated insulin disappearance from the blood in man before and after renal transplantation. The disappearance rate of [131] I-insulin injected in tracer amounts was significantly slower prior to receipt of the allograft. After

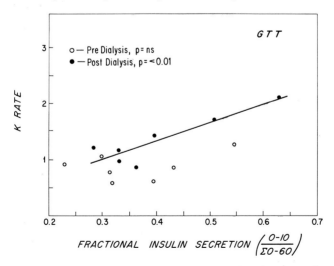

Fig. 3. Correlation between 10-minute fractional estimated insulin secretion [16] and K rate in uremic individuals before and after dialysis. A significant correlation is noted in post-dialysis uremic individuals.

transplantation, disappearance rates approached normal. Silvers and his associates [25] have also demonstrated delayed insulin degradation in patients with renal failure, and it is logically assumed that the loss of functioning renal mass leads directly to the attenuated insulin disappearance. This, however, does not explain all available data. For instance, adequate hemodialysis shortens the prolonged half-life of insulin in the blood in these uremic individuals. Figure 4 illustrates this point. Exogenous insulin was administered to patients prior to dialysis and was given again after a period of adequate hemodialysis. Insulin half-life was significantly shortened in well-dialyzed individuals even though 6 of the 7 patients were anephric [10]. Therefore, loss of renal mass cannot totally explain the attenuated insulin metabolism, and uremia per se must have some effect.

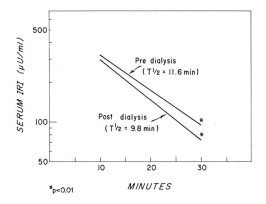

Fig. 4.   Insulin disappearance during insulin tolerance testing in 7 patients—6 of whom were anephric—was more rapid after adequate hemodialysis.

In summary, in insulin metabolism in chronic reanal failure, secretion is adequate in amount, although the pancreatic response is somewhat slowed. Insulin degradation rate is slow, and the residence time of insulin in the blood is prolonged. This prolonged degradation rate of insulin may be due in part to a loss of functioning renal mass. Adequate hemodialysis tends to speed insulin degradation, however, implying that the uremic state is also influential.

Most investigators agree that the peripheral tissues are somewhat insensitive to the action of insulin in chronic renal failure [4-6,8-16]. Hutchings and co-workers [7] found only 2 out of 10 uremic individuals who exhibited an abnormal glucose-insulin tolerance test. Most other investigators, however [5,12,13], have noted that blood glucose falls to a lower percentage of fasting after the intravenous administration of insulin in normal subjects than in uremic patients. Horton and associates [14] have shown a slowed glucose disappearance rate in uremic subjects after the intravenous administration of insulin. Furthermore, fasting hyperinsulinemia is usually present in azotemic patients, both before and after adequate hemodialysis, and Bagdade and co-workers [26] have shown that fasting hyperinsulinemia correlates with insensitivity of peripheral tissues to insulin.

Hampers and associates [13] demonstrated some improvement in insulin responsiveness with hemodialysis. Table 3 shows glucose K rates during intravenous glucose-insulin tolerance testing and during insulin tolerance testing, before and after 2 weeks of hemodialysis. Statistically significant (by sign or Wilcoxan test) improvement followed hemodialysis in both instances indicating that therapy improved the sensitivity of the peripheral tissues to the action of insulin.

Table 3

Glucose K Rates* During Glucose-Insulin Tolerance Tests and Insulin Tolerance Tests in Uremic Individuals Before and After Dialysis

	Glucose-Insulin Test		Insulin Tolerance Test	
Patient	Predialysis	Postdialysis	Predialysis	Postdialysis
1			0.92	4.40
2	2.73	2.28	2.62	3.09
3	1.55	2.68	2.71	3.12
4	1.34	3.13	2.10	3.24
5	1.24	1.99	1.45	2.11
6	1.27	2.03	1.51	2.67
7	1.54	3.12	2.23	2.05
Mean	1.61	2.54	1.93	2.95
	$< .05$		$< .05$	

*Exponential disappearance rate multiplied by -100.

Westervelt [27,28] has measured fluxes of glucose, potassium, lactate, and inorganic phosphate in the forearms of uremic individuals after infusing standardized amounts of insulin into their brachial arteries. Glucose, potassium, and phosphate uptakes are diminished and lactate output is less in these patients than in normal subjects—findings which suggest that the uremic patient's forearm is more resistant to the action of insulin than that of his normal counterpart. Spitz and co-workers [11] have demonstrated an attenuated fall in serum phosphate during oral glucose tolerance testing. Similarly, during intravenous tolbutamide tolerance testing and after intravenous insulin infusion, serum phosphate fell significantly less in uremic patients than in normal individuals. Plasma-free fatty acids, while higher in uremics than in normals, was lowered to comparable levels in both groups after oral glucose. These findings further suggest that the primary site of insulin resistance may reside in muscle rather than in adipose tissue [11].

Some investigators [6,29] have felt that the glucose intolerance complicating chronic renal failure may be due to impaired glyco-genesis—a hypothesis based primarily upon the observation that the blood sugar response of uremic individuals to glucagon was less than that found in normals. Phosphate responses were similar to those observed in normal individuals during glucose tolerance testing, and uremic patients experienced a greater incidence of symptomatic hypo-glycemia after insulin infusion. Furthermore, liver glycogen was reduced in rats made uremic by partial nephrectomy. Other investigators [5,13], however, have observed normal glucagon responsiveness in azotemia, and the hypoglycemia found after insulin administration may be explained by a prolonged insulin half-life as well as by glycogen depletion. Boucot and associates [30,31] have demonstrated normal hepatic glycogen content in uremic rats, and Spitz and co-workers [11] have shown abnormal serum phosphate responses to oral glucose. Lindner et al [1] have also suggested that glycogenesis may be impaired in renal failure. This conclusion was based on the observation that the respiratory quotient was normal in uremic patients. Other investigators [10,16], however, have noted that the response of the respiratory quotient is flat or minimal after a glucose load in undialyzed uremic individuals. This abnormality is improved by hemodialysis so that the respiratory quotient increases normally after carbohydrate administration. Based on all available evidence, it seems unlikely that the liver is the primary site of the abnormality.

Elevated levels of plasma growth hormone described in chronic renal failure [14] could cause the abnormal glucose response. But abnormalities in growth hormone do not correlate well with abnormalities in glucose metabolism [14]. Further, Tchobroutsky and co-workers [32] have demonstrated that the pattern of growth hormone and glucagon secretion is normal in well-nourished patients with chronic renal failure. Nonetheless, the patients had glucose intolerance and prolonged insulin secretion.

Hyperparathyroidism is a well-established complication of chronic renal failure. The report of Kim and co-workers [33] that insulin resistance may coexist with primary hyperparathyroidism is of great interest in this regard. Fasting plasma-insulin concentrations and insulin responses to administered glucose and tolbutamide were significantly greater in individuals with primary hyperparathyroidism prior to removal of adenomas than they were after surgery. This hyperinsulinemia was not associated with altered glucose metabolism, but the glucose-lowering action of intravenous insulin was slightly impaired before surgery. Parenteral parathormone administered to normal individuals induced mild hypercalcemia and hypophosphatemia and reproduced the augmented insulin responses to oral glucose. The authors concluded that hypercalcemia sustains a form of endogenous insulin resistance that requires augmented insulin secretion to maintain glucose homeostasis, but they were unable to evaluate the direct role of parathyroid hormone in this setting. The pattern of this form of carbohydrate intolerance is similar to that observed in uremia. In this regard, Lindall and co-workers [34] observed that the insulin responses of dialyzed patients were normal if hyperparathyroidism was absent but were increased if it was present. These insulin responses returned toward normal after the hyperplastic glands were removed. No difference in K-rate between the two groups was observed, however. The possible interaction of hyperparathyroidism and glucose intolerance in chronic renal failure obviously requires further investigation.

It is attractive to speculate that dialysis improves carbohydrate metabolism by removing some dialyzable insulin antagonist. Unfortunately, such an antagonist has not been found. Davidson and co-workers [35] employed an insulin-stimulated rat hemidiaphragm assay specifically designed to measure insulin antagonism. The serum of patients with chronic renal failure was examined before and after repeated hemodialysis. No evidence for a dialyzable antagonist could be found, even though glucose tolerance improved in every patient.

It is not clear whether insulin insensitivity is due to tissue resistance to the action of insulin per se or to some abnormality distal to the site of insulin action. Dzurik and Krajci-Lazary [36] have shown that rat diaphragms incubated in the serum of patients with renal insufficiency utilize less glucose than diaphragms incubated in the serum of normal volunteers. Since there was no difference in oxygen consumption, metabolic substrates other than glucose must have been metabolized. While diaphragms incubated in normal serum tended to synthesize glycogen, diaphragms incubated in uremic serum utilized it. If lactate or α-ketoglutarate were added to the media, control diaphragms still released these substances, while diaphragms incubated in uremic sera took them up. The data suggest an abnormality in either the transmembrane transfer of glucose or the metabolism of this substance somewhere in the Embden-Meyerhoff pathway. This assay procedure is not, strictly speaking, comparable to that of Davidson and co-workers [35], since the latter technique employed insulin stimulation. Dzurik's data suggest that there may be a substance in uremic plasma that blocks glucose utilization, but the substance is not necessarily an antagonist of insulin per se.

Other studies examining the more distal end of the Embden-Meyerhoff pathway may shed light on possible abnormalities. Patients suffering from chronic renal failure generally exhibit a low blood-lactate concentration [37]. Following intravenous administration of lactate, however, the blood-lactate concentration increases more than it does in normal subjects, and lactate levels return to baseline more slowly than in healthy volunteers. Gluconcogenesis from pyruvate, fructose, and α-ketoglutarate was studied in rat kidney slices in the presence of uremic or normal serum [38]. Uremic serum effected a 42 percent inhibition of glucose formation from pyruvate. No inhibition in glycogen formation from fructose was found, excluding the possibility of an inhibition of gluconeogenesis proximal to the site of conversion of fructose-6-phosphate to glucose. Glucose production from α-ketoglutarate was inhibited by 17 percent in uremic serum. This differential inhibition of 42 versus 17 percent suggests that there may be some abnormality in pyruvate metabolism at the level of pyruvate carboxylase which is the enzyme that converts pyruvate to oxalacetate [38].

Finally, the studies of Renner and Heintz [39] have suggested other glycolytic abnormalities that may be independent of insulin. They found, for instance, that glucose utilization via the hexose-monophosphate shunt in erythrocytes incubated in a uremic milieu is 4 to 5 times higher than utilization in normal erythrocytes. This suggests some abnormality in the Embden-Meyerhoff pathway. Further, phosphofructokinase activity is low in uremic erythrocytes. It is becoming increasingly clear, therefore, that abnormalities of glucose utilization distal to the site of insulin action may well exist in uremia. Furthermore, these anomalies may result from certain toxic serum factors that accumulate in uremia. Renner and Heintz [39], for instance, point out that phenylacrylic acid and phenylpyruvic acid have been shown to inhibit glucose utilization and glucose formation in brain and kidney cortex slices, respectively, and these substances have been isolated from extracts of hemodialysate.

The literature to date is consistent with the thesis that glucose intolerance associated with uremia is caused by peripheral tissue insensitivity to insulin, perhaps not secondary to insulin antagonism per se. Insulin secretion is normal in amount but initial pancreatic release is somewhat slowed. The onset of hemodialysis is associated with augmentation of insulin secretion in uremic patients to greater levels than are observed in matched normal controls. Peripheral glucose utilization also seems to be improved by hemodialysis. The combined effect of augmented insulin secretion and improved insulin sensitivity after hemodialysis improves, but usually does not totally normalize, carbohydrate tolerance. Some available data suggest that the peripheral malutilization of glucose may be due to inhibition of metabolism —perhaps by toxic or competing plasma factors—at sites distal to the action of insulin.

LIPID METABOLISM

Even though abnormalities in lipid metabolism coincident with uremia have been appreciated for some years [40-42], relatively little information is available on the metabolism of fat in patients with chronic renal failure. Serum cholesterol levels have been variously reported as high [41], low [40], and normal [42-44]. Fasting-free fatty acids may be normal, but are frequently elevated [11] and tend to fall normally during glucose tolerance testing [11]. Conversely, serum triglycerides are abnormally elevated in most uremic patients [45-48], and this probably constitutes the most characteristic abnormality of the blood-lipid profile in individuals with chronic renal failure.

A recent lipid survey was performed at the Peter Bent Brigham Hospital on 77 patients ranging in age from 12 to 70 years [49]. All suffered from chronic renal failure and had been on dialysis for varying periods of time. The results of this survey are shown in Table 4. As

Table 4

Lipid Survey in Patients with Renal Failure

Duration of Dialysis	Number	Average Age (yr)	Cholesterol* (mg/100 ml)	Triglycerides* (ml/100 ml)
0 (uremic)	17	37	215 ± 12.2	135 ± 32.9
1 wk–6 mo	14	36	215 ± 15.3	165 ± 18.1
6 mo–1 yr	25	38	223 ± 10.5	259 ± 36.4
1–2 yr	14	46	247 ± 14.8	375 ± 55.4
2–3 yr	5	42	221 ± 19.1	269 ± 62.0
> 3 yr	2	37	199 ± 20.1	320 ± 46.4

*Mean ± SEM.

noted by the standard errors shown, wide variation in serum cholesterol was observed. Nonetheless, if one assumes the upper limit of normal for serum cholesterol to be 250 mg/100 ml for individuals under 40 and 300 mg/100 ml for patients over 40, only 24 percent and 7.5 percent of patients under and over 40 years of age, respectively, exhibited abnormal values. There appears to be no distinct correlation between serum cholesterol and length of dialysis therapy. A much greater incidence of elevated serum triglycerides was observed. Seventy-one percent of individuals under the age of 40 (normal = 150 mg/100 ml) and 64 percent of individuals over that age (normal = 190 mg/100 ml) had abnormally high values. Although statistical significance was not achieved, there may be a trend toward increasing triglyceride levels with increasing duration of hemodialysis therapy. If so, this trend may level off at the 1- to 2-year period. Twenty-seven lipoprotein electrophoreses were performed. Of these, only 6 were clearly normal. Three others showed a slight increase in the prebeta fraction and were considered borderline normal. The remaining 18 were clearly abnormal by Fredrickson's classification [50]. One patient could be classified as type 2, one as type 3, and one as type 5, while 15 patients were considered typical of type 4 hyperlipoproteinemia.

These considerations may have important prognostic and therapeutic implications for patients with chronic renal failure who are being maintained with hemodialysis. The association of arteriosclerotic cardiovascular disease with hyperlipoproteinemia in general, and Type 4 hyperlipoproteinemia in particular, is well established [50,51]. These observations are important since the greatest contributing factors to mortality in individuals undergoing chronic hemodialysis are related to heart disease and arteriosclerotic vascular disease [52-55].

The most rational insight into the potential mechanisms responsible for the high incidence of hyperglyceridemia has been provided by Bagdade and co-workers [45-48]. In general, increased concentrations of these substances may be due primarily to increased synthesis, diminished removal, or a combination of these effects. Bagdade and associates have observed reduced lipoprotein lipase activity in the serum of individuals with chronic renal failure and have noted that hemodialysis appears to improve this abnormality [48]. Insulin has been shown to be necessary for maintaining normal tissue lipoprotein lipase levels and normal triglyceride assimilation [56,57]. Hence, insulin resistance may influence the etiology of this abnormality.

These same investigators have shown that elevations of fasting immunoreactive insulin may well reflect a state of relative insulin resistance [26]. Fasting hyperinsulinemia, a characteristic finding in patients with chronic renal failure [11,15,48], is improved—but may not be normalized—by hemodialysis [15].

Fasting-immunoreactive insulin levels are correlated with fasting levels of serum triglyceride in nonuremic subjects [45-48,56]. This observation suggests that hyperinsulinemia is associated with an increased hepatic output of glycerides. Plasma glycerides also correlate well with fasting immunoreactive insulin in uremic individuals [45-48], and such elevated serum glycerides may reflect hyperinsulinemia, which is in turn a result of the resistance of peripheral tissues to the action of insulin. Fasting triglycerides, fasting immunoreactive insulin, and glucose tolerance all tend to improve when patients are adequately hemodialyzed [48]. Hyperglyceridemia may be carbohydrate inducible [50], and one might theorize that repeated exposure to carbohydrate-containing dialysate could aggravate the abnormality. Hubner et al [58] studied the effects of glucose-free dialysate on plasma-lipid profiles and were unable to demonstrate any significant lowering of triglyceride levels by this treatment.

The characteristic hyperglyceridemia of chronic renal failure may then be due to a combination of effects. First, the insensitivity of peripheral tissues to insulin may lead to a relative hyperinsulinemic state. This, in turn, may stimulate the hepatic output of glycerides. Reduced lipoprotein lipase activity—perhaps also due to relative insulin resistance—could contribute to the abnormality. As noted previously, the presence of a dialyzable insulin antagonist seems unlikely [35] and resistance to the action of insulin may be due to an intracellular defect in the glycolytic cycle distal to the cell wall site of insulin action.

PROTEIN METABOLISM

Elevations in blood-urea concentration have been considered the hallmark of uremia. While the uremic syndrome is a constellation of various effects, the breakdown products of protein metabolism or aberrations in protein metabolism are of prime importance. Unfortunately, relatively little is known about the mechanisms by which protein metabolism is altered in uremia, and even the nature of the aberrations that do occur is obscure.

It is not surprising that dietary therapy aimed at lowering the nitrogenous load has received considerable attention and found place in the treatment of chronic renal failure [59]. Although earlier attempts were complicated by symptoms of general malnutrition, recent efforts have yielded more gratifying results [60]. Nonetheless, the benefits of dietary treatment of necessity are limited [61].

Farr and Smadel showed that rats with renal failure from nephrotoxic nephritis survived more frequently if dietary protein was restricted than if a high-protein diet was allowed [62]. Rose and Dekker [63] administered urea labeled with isotopic nitrogen to two groups of rats. One was maintained on a diet containing essential amino acids, while the other received casein as dietary protein. The distribution of isotope in the carcasses of these animals suggested that urea nitrogen could be used for the synthesis of nonessential amino acids and protein if essential amino acids were provided in the diet. The studies of Josephson and colleagues [64] have suggested that the nitrogen from ^{15}N urea can be incorporated into the muscle nonessential amino acids of patients with renal failure. The patterns of incorporation were similar to those of a normal patient except that histadine was not labeled in uremics as it was in normals. This observation and those of Giordano [65] suggest that histadine may be an essential amino acid in patients with chronic renal failure.

Isotopic studies by Shear [66] have shown that net protein synthesis is increased in the liver and heart but decreased in skeletal muscle in bilaterally nephrectomized rats. He found that lysine may shift from muscle to liver in association with these changes in protein synthesis. Uremia also altered tissue levels of other amino acids and liver to blood concentration ratios tended to increase for essential but not for nonessential amino acids. The data suggest that acute uremia may selectively alter tissue composition and protein synthesis in different organs and may modify in different ways the metabolism of individual amino acids.

Giordano [65] has also postulated that uremic man as well as laboratory animals can reutilize urea nitrogen for the synthesis of nonessential amino acids. This postulate has been confirmed by isotopic studies [65,68]. Four uremic subjects were given diets containing normal or low amounts of protein with essential amino acids as nitrogen sources [68]. Urea tagged with ^{15}N or ^{14}C were added to the diets. Plasma albumin was separated from blood drawn approximately 24 hours after the administration of the isotope and was hydrolyzed to component amino acids. The 18 amino acids studied all contained significant amounts of radioactivity, but glutamic acid, alanine, aspartic acid, serine, and glycine were labeled to a significantly greater extent than others.

Balance studies with low-protein diets (approximately 20 gm) containing adequate amounts of essential amino acids have been introduced into the therapy of chronic renal failure [60,69-72] and have been associated with positive nitrogen balance. Some uremic symptoms—

especially nausea and other gastrointestinal symptoms—are relieved and patients generally acquire a feeling of well-being. There is, however, no conclusive evidence that patients maintained on diet therapy alone live longer than they would if diet therapy had never been instituted, and terminally they become acidotic and succumb to classical symptoms of uremia [72].

Other investigators have suggested that more protein may be required to induce positive nitrogen balance in undialyzed individuals with chronic renal failure. Kopple and co-workers [73,74] studied patients with chronic renal failure on diets containing approximately 20 to 40 gm of high biological value protein. They concluded that there was no significant difference in the level of symptomatic improvement between these diets, and both groups of patients did well. Patients on a lower protein diet, however, complained about the severe protein restriction. Further, balance studies revealed that while nitrogen balance improved in patients on the 20-gm protein diet, it generally remained slightly negative. In contrast, nitrogen balance invariably became positive when more protein was administered. On the other hand, patients with low urea clearances became ill when they received dietary protein amounting to approximately 1 gm/kg [73].

These authors have also assessed protein requirements in patients undergoing chronic hemodialysis [75]. Patients received either 0.75 or 1.25 gm of protein per kilogram of body weight. Predialysis blood urea nitrogen correlated with average daily protein intake, increasing as expected with higher protein intakes. Serum albumin levels increased significantly in both groups, suggesting that previous dietary intake may have been inadequate. The lower protein diet was associated with a slightly positive and the high protein diet with a more strongly positive nitrogen balance. Both diets were associated with a gain in body weight, but the gain was more striking with greater protein intake. Hematocrit did not change significantly in either group. Patients consuming more protein tended to exhibit somewhat more "uremic symptomatology" than those on the lower protein diet. The experience of these investigators, as well as that of others, has been reviewed recently [76]. The data suggest that patients undergoing chronic hemodialysis be fed a diet containing at least 35 calories/kg of body weight and at least 0.8 to 0.9 gm/kg of protein, of which 0.63 gm/kg should be of high biological value. These suggestions are in good agreement with those of other authors [77].

Bianchi and co-workers [78] studied albumin metabolism in uremic patients on low protein diets which contained at least 18 gm of high biological value protein per day. Tracer kinetics revealed that the intravascular albumin mass was normal, but that there was a marked reduction in the total body albumin pool and extravascular albumin. The catabolic rate of serum albumin was within normal limits. Bischel and colleagues [79], on the other hand, demonstrated mild hypoalbuminemia in chronic hemodialysis patients who received 50 to 60 gm protein per day and were dialyzed twice weekly on a Kiil dialyzer. Radioiodinated serum albumin turnover studies revealed accelerated turnover in patients whose serum albumin concentration was less than 3 gm/100 ml. Albumin loss could not be totally explained by loss as a result of hemodialysis or proteinuria. The authors postulated gastrointestinal protein loss in this patients, but were unable to prove this hypothesis.

Other investigators [80] have found normal albumin turnover rates in patients on chronic hemodialysis. In general, these patients consumed approximately 80 gm of protein per day and dialysis was performed three times weekly. Serum albumin concentrations increased when patients were placed on adequate hemodialysis. The authors found elevated plasma volumes, normal serum albumin concentrations, and elevated intravascular albumin and total exchangeable albumin. Albumin half-lives and turnover rates were within normal limits. Adequate protein intake and adequate hemodialysis, then, appears to be associated with normal albumin kinetics. Total body albumin is increased, probably as a result of the increased plasma volume which must by necessity accompany the anemia of chronic renal failure.

Amino acids are the building blocks for proteins. There has been recent interest in the metabolism of these substances in patients with chronic renal failure and in patients undergoing chronic hemodialysis. Gulyassy and associates [81-83] have pointed out that while total α-amino-nitrogen in the serum of patients with chronic renal failure may be normal or elevated [84], marked derangements in the serum concentration of various amino acids may exist. For example, aspartic acid, citrulline, cystine, 1- and 3-methylhistidine, proline, and taurine seem to be significantly *elevated* in patients with chronic renal failure and in those undergoing chronic hemodialysis. Hemodialysis does not seem to normalize these elevated values. While the high levels of both 3-methylhistidine and cystine are reduced by a period of hemodialysis, the levels of these substances remain significantly elevated. Renal transplantation, on the other hand, effectively reduces plasma concentrations [82]. The consequences of maintaining high levels of these amino acids are not clear.

Conversely, the plasma concentrations of some amino acids, such as α-amino-butyic acid, histidine, serine, tyrosine, isoleucine, leucine, lysine, threonine, trypophan and valine, are significantly *reduced*. The last 6 substances mentioned are essential amino acids. The causes for and consequences of these reductions are also unclear. Inadequate dietary intake may certainly play a role. However, acute oral loading with radioactive-labeled tryptophan in patients with chronic renal failure yields a significantly delayed and blunted plasma radioactivity curve when compared to normal. For a given volume of distribution, such an observation could be due either to attentuated absorption into or augmented removal from the serum. Current data do not unequivocally dissect these possible effects. Furthermore, if certain amino acids are removed from the serum more rapidly in patients with renal failure than in normals, the methods by which this is effected are not clear. Augmented plasma clearance, for example, could be due to more rapid renal clearance, altered hepatic clearance, or some other as yet undefined mechanism. While none of these considerations is currently resolved, the relative renal clearance (expressed as a percentage of creatinine clearance) is much higher for all amino acids in patients with chronic renal failure than in normal individuals [83]. Tyrosine, for example, is generally cleared at a rate less than 1 percent of the creatinine clearance. In patients with chronic renal failure, its clearance may approximate 20 percent of creatinine clearance. While these figures are impressive, the total excretion of amino acids (e.g., milligrams per day) generally would not differ from those observed in normal patients.

Hemodialysis does not seem to predictably alter the plasma concentration of amino acids which are initially low in chronic renal failure. Patients thus continue to show depressed levels of these substances despite adequate hemodialysis and good control of clinical uremia. Two exceptions are isoleucine and threonine, which approach but do not achieve normal levels after the commencement of hemodialysis. Again, the causes and consequences of these observed abnormalities remains to be defined.

Some insights can be gleaned from the literature, however. Tryptophan, for example, is bound to serum albumin [85]. As noted, serum tryptophan levels are generally lower than normal in patients with chronic renal failure. In spite of this observation, the ratio of bound to unbound tryptophan in the serum of patients with chronic renal failure is below normal [86]. Presumably, some as yet undefined substance competes successfully with tryptophan for albumin-binding sites. A relatively greater fraction of tryptophan is then unbound and is free and available for clearance or metabolism. This concept of reduced protein binding of a substance leading to augmented metabolism has precedent in the pharmacologic literature as it pertains to chronic renal failure [87].

Impaired synthesis may also cause reduced plasma concentrations of various amino acids. Serum tyrosine, for example, is generally low, while serum phenylalanine concentrations are generally high or normal [81,83]. Plasma phenylalanine to tyrosine ratios are high, and isotopic studies suggest that the oxidation of tyrosine in patients with chronic renal failure is normal [88]. The combined observations of high phenylalanine to tyrosine ratio, low tyrosine concentration, and normal tyrosine degradation suggest that in uremic patients the conversion of phenylalanine to tyrosine by phenylalanine hydroxylase may be abnormal. Phenylalanine hydroxylase is known to exist in the liver, pancreas, and kidney [89]. In general, an abnormal conversion could be due to an inhibitor of phenylalanine hydroxylase, nonavailability of circulating phenylalanine, or reduced amounts of available phenylalanine hydroxylase in the body. Since the ratio of phenylalanine to tyrosine in the plasma becomes more abnormal with greater reductions in glomerular filtration rate [88], it is possible that the loss of renal phenylalanine hydroxylase which attends reduction in functioning renal mass may contribute to these abnormalities of tyrosine and phenylalanine metabolism. Again, there is precedent for this concept in the pharmacologic literature. Insulin degradation, for example, is slowed in chronic renal failure due, at least in part, to reduced renal mass [25]. Further, the final hydroxylation of vitamin D, resulting in its biologically active form, likely occurs in the kidneys. Reduction in renal mass and metabolic activity may attenuate this normal conversion [90], contributing to the well-appreciated abnormalities in calcium homeostasis that complicate chronic renal failure.

To date we can only speculate about the abnormalities of intermediary metabolism that complicate chronic renal failure. It is clear, however, that hemodialysis in its present form does not restore body metabolism to normal. A better understanding of these metabolic aberrations is obviously germane to improving the long-term course of patients suffering from chronic renal failure.

MISCELLANEOUS TOPICS

Many aspects of endocrine function in chronic renal failure have not been thoroughly evaluated. Reviews of this topic are not generally available and, unlike mineral metabolism, hypertension, and anemia, endocrinology is not usually considered a subtopic of uremia.

Obviously, the endocrine system is integrally related to other aspects of chronic renal failure and, as such, discussions of some aspects of endocrine function are scattered throughout these pages. Parathyroid abnormalities, for instance, are covered in the section on the skeletal system (Chap. 10). The renin-angiotensin-adrenal axis is discussed in the chapter on hypertension (Chap. 5), and growth hormone and insulin are covered elsewhere in this chapter.

There is a general lack of available information regarding the thyroid in uremia. Iodine kinetics [91] have revealed increased plasma levels of inorganic iodine and reduced thyroidal iodine clearance. The 24-hour absolute uptake of iodine, however, is increased. Urinary excretion of iodine and renal iodine clearance is decreased, and these factors—combined with an adequate dietary intake—probably lead to the increased plasma-iodine levels which in turn contribute to the reduced thyroidal clearance. Ramirez and co-workers [92] have observed an enlarged thyroid gland in a substantial number of their patients. At 2, 6, and 24 hours, ^{131}I uptake tended to be low, while levels of thyroxine-binding globulin, triiodothyronine, and thyroid-stimulating hormone were normal. Triiodothyronine resin uptake was also normal, but serum thyroxine, while normal in most, was low in some patients. Free plasma iodides were unfortunately not determined. The authors concluded that thyroid function was generally normal in their dialysis patients despite thyromegaly. Their results demonstrating borderline low or low ^{131}I uptake and normal serum thyroxine could conceivably be due to expansion of the body iodide pool. Further, their incidence of thyromegaly has not been observed in the country at large [93].

Review of patients on whom thyroid function studies have been performed at the Peter Bent Brigham Hospital [49] reveals widely disparate results. Marked variation in resin triiodothyronine uptake, protein-bound iodine, free thyroxine, and triiodothyronine was observed in patients both before and after the initiation of hemodialysis. These individuals were clinically euthyroid, however. Twenty-four hour ^{131}I uptake, on the other hand, was normal and appeared to be the most consistently reliable estimator of thyroid function. The confusing results of thyroid function tests notwithstanding, the thyroid gland is generally considered to be normal in patients with chronic renal failure and in patients undergoing chronic hemodialysis.

As uremia progresses, loss of libido is very common in both sexes. In women of child-bearing age, menstruation commonly ceases and men may become impotent. A period of adequate hemodialysis *may* result in a return of menstrual function to women and potency to men.

Testosterone levels in men [49] tend to be low prior to the initiation of dialysis. After a period of adequate hemodialysis, however, levels tend to rise into the normal range. Furthermore, fertility may return to the male dialysis patient, and reports of men impregnating their spouses are available [94]. It is distinctly unusual for a female dialysis patient to conceive and deliver a child. Only one such report is available [95]. Endogenous creatinine clearance in this patient was 9.2 ml/min at the time hemodialysis was initiated, and this relatively good residual renal function may have contributed to the successful outcome of the pregnancy. While other verbal reports of pregnancies in dialysis patients are available [96], these pregnancies usually result in an early spontaneous abortion.

Gynecomastia, relatively common in patients undergoing hemodialysis [97-99], frequently occurs soon after the initiation of therapy. The hypertrophied breast tissue is frequently tender and may be present either bilaterally or on only one side. Poor sexual function, small testes, and impaired spermatogenesis frequently accompany the syndrome. The precise cause of this occurrence is unknown, but it is compared to the refeeding gynecomastia reported to occur in men after incarceration in prison camps.

REFERENCES

1. Lindner, G.C., Hiller, A., Van Slyke, D.D.: Carbohydrate metabolism in nephritis. J Clin Invest 1:247, 1925.
2. Williams, J.R., Humphries, E.M.: Clinical significance of blood sugar in nephritis and other diseases. Arch Intern Med 23:537, 1919.
3. Zubrod, C.G., Eversole, S.L., Dana, G.W.: Amelioration of diabetes and striking rarity of acidosis in patients with Kimmelstiel-Wilson lesions. N Engl J Med 245:518, 1951.
4. Briggs, J.D., Buchanan, K.D., Luke, R.G., et al: Role of insulin in glucose intolerance inuraemia. Lancet 1:462, 1967.
5. Cerletty, J.M., Enbring, N.H.: Azotemia and glucose intolerance. Ann Intern Med 66:1097, 1967.
6. Cohen, B.D.: Abnormal carbohydrate metabolism in renal disease. Ann Intern Med 57:204, 1962.
7. Hutchings, R.H., Hegstrom, R.M., Scribner, B.H.: Glucose intolerance in patients on long-term intermittent dialysis. Ann Intern Med 65:276, 1966.
8. Perkoff, G.T., Thomas, C.L., Newton, J.D., et al: Mechanism of impaired glucose tolerance in uremia and experimental hyperazotemia. Diabetes 7:375, 1958.

9. Hampers, C.L., Soeldner, J.S., Gleason, R.E., et al: Insulin-glocuse relationships in uremia. Am J Clin Nutr 21:414, 1967.

10. Hampers,C.L., Lowrie, E.G., Soeldner, J.S., et al: The effect of uremia upon glucose metabolism. Arch Intern Med 126:868, 1970.

11. Spitz, I.M., Rubenstein, A.H., Bersohn, I., et al: Carbohydrate metabolism in renal disease. Q J Med 39:301, 1970.

12. Westervelt, F.B., Schreiner, G.E.: The carbohydrate intolerance of uremic patients. Ann Intern Med 57:266, 1962.

13. Hampers, C.L., Soeldner, J.S.,Doak, P.B., et al: Effect of chronic renal failure and hemodialysis on carbohydrate metabolism. J Clin Invest 45: 1719, 1966.

14. Horton, E.S., Johnson, C., Lebovits, H.E.: Carbohydrate metabolism in uremia. Ann Intern Med 68:63, 1968.

15. Lowrie, E.G., Soeldner, J.S., Hampers, C.L., et al: Glucose metabolism and insulin secretion in uremia, prediabetic and normal subjects. J Lab Clin Med 76:603, 1970.

16. Hampers, C.L., Lowrie, E.G., Soeldner, J.S., et al: Uremia andcarbohydrate metabolism, in Kluthe, R., Berlyne, G., Burton, B. (eds): Uremia: An International Congress in Pathogenesis, Diagnosis and Therapy. Stuttgart, Georg Theime Verlag, 1972, p 173.

17. Alfrey, A.C., Sussman, K.E., Holmes, J.H.: Changes in glucose and insulin metabolism induced by dialysis in patients with chronic uremia. Metabolism 16:733, 1967.

18. Sagild, V.: Glucose tolerance in acute ischemic renal failure. Acta Med Scand 172:405, 1962.

19. Speigel, G., Bleicher, S.J., Goldberg, M., et al: The effect of potassium on the impaired glucose tolerance in chronic uremia. Metabolism 16: 581, 1967.

20. Hampers, C.L., Zollinger, R.M., Skillman, J.J., et al: Hemodynamic and body composition changes following bilateral nephrectomy in chronic renal failure. Circulation 40:367, 1969.

21. Boddy, K., Kings, P.C., Lindsay, R.M., et al: Exchangeable and total body potassium in patients with chronic renal failure. Br Med J 1:140, 1972.

22. Garcia, M.J., Soeldner, J.S., Gleason, R.E., et al: Relationship of blood glucose (BG) and serum immunoreactive insulin (IRI)during repeated intravenous glucose tolerance tests (IVGTT) in normals. J Clin Invest 45:1010, 1966.

23. Rubenstein, A.H., Spitz, I.: Role of the kidney in insulin metabolism and excretion. Diabetes 17:161, 1968.

24. O'Brien, J.P., Sharpe, A.R.: The influence of renal disease on the insulin I[131] disappearance curve in man. Metabolism 16:76, 1967.

25. Silvers, A., Swenson, R.S., Farquhar, J.W., et al: Derivation of a three compartmental model disappearance of plasma insulin I[131] in man. J Clin Invest 48:1461, 1969.

26. Bagdade, J.D., Bierman, E.L., Porte, D., Jr.: The significance of basal insulin levels in the evaluation of the insulin response to glucose in diabetic subjects. J Clin Invest 46:1549, 1967.

27. Westervelt, F.B., Jr.: Abnormal carbohydrate metabolism in uremia. Am J Clin Nutr 21:423, 1968.
28. Westervelt, F.B., Jr.: Insulin effect in uremia. J Lab Clin Med 74:79, 1969.
29. Cohen, B.D., Horowitz, H.L.: Carbohydrate metabolism in uremia: Ihhibition of phosphate release. Am J Clin Nutr 21:407, 1968.
30. Boucot, N.G.,Guild, W.R., Merrill, J.P.: Carbohydrate metabolism in rats with acute uremia. Am J Physiol 192:30, 1958.
31. Boucot, N.G., Nurser, E.K., Merrill, J.P.: Carbohydrate metabolism in rats with chronic uremia. Am J Physiol 198:797, 1960.
32. Tchobroutsky, G., Rosselin, G., Assan, R., et al: Glucose intolerance in uraemia. II. Plasma growth hormone and glucagon values. Diabetologia 5:25, 1969.
33. Kim, H., Kalkhoff, R.K., Costrini, N.V., et al: Plasma insulin disturbances in primary hyperparathyroidism. J Clin Invest 50:2596, 1971.
34. Lindall, A., Carmena, R., Cohen, S., et al: Insulin hypersecretion in patients on chronic hemodialysis. Role of parathyroids. J Clin Endocrinol Metab 32:653, 1971.
35. Davidson, M.B., Lowrie, E.G., Hampers, C.L.: Lack of dialyzable insulin antagonist in uremia. Metabolism 18:387, 1969.
36. Dzurik, R., Krajci-Lazary, B.: The effect of uremia serum on carbohydrate metabolism in rat diaphragm. Experientia 23:798, 1967.
37. Dzurik, R.: Lactate utilization in chronic uremia. Vnitr Lek 15:3, 1969.
38. Dzurik, R., Simoncic, E.: Localization of the inhibition of gluconeogenesis in kidney slices by uremic serum. Med Exp 18:135, 1968.
39. Renner, D., Heintz, R.: The inhibition of certain steps of glucose degradation in uremia, in Kluthe, R., Berlyne, G., Burton, B. (eds), Uremia: An International Congress in Pathogenesis, Diagnosis and Therapy. Stuttgart, Georg Theime Verlag, 1972, p 195.
40. Ashe, B.J., Bruger, M.: The cholesterol content of the plasma in chronic nephritis and retention uremia. Am J Med Sci 186:670, 1933.
41. Winkler, A.M., Durlacher, S.H., Hoff, H.E., et al: Changes in lipid content of serum and of liver following bilateral renal ablation or ureteral ligation. J Exp Med 77:473, 1943.
42. Ludewig, S., Chanutin, A.: Experimental renal insufficiency produced by partial nephrectomy. Arch Intern Med 61:354, 1938.
43. Sunderman, W.: Studies in serum electrolytes: XX. Renal insufficiency. N Y State J Med 53:57, 1953.
44. DiLuzio, W.R., Houck, C.R.: The role of the kidney in the etiology of renal hyperlipemia. J Clin Invest 35:1381, 1956.
45. Bagdade, J.D., Porte, D., Jr., Bierman, E.L.: Hypertriglyceridemia: a metabolic consequence of chronic renal failure. N Engl J Med 279: 181, 1968.
46. Bagdade, J.D.: Lipemia, a sequela of chronic renal failure and hemodialysis. Am J Clin Nutr 21:426, 1968.
47. Bagdade, J.D., Porte, D., Curtis, F.K., et al: Uremic lipemia: an unrecognized abnormality on triglyceride synthesis and removal. Trans Assoc Am Physicians 81:190, 1968.

48. Bagdade, J.D.: Uremic lipemia: an unrecognized abnormality in tri- glyceride production and removal. Arch Intern Med 7:875, 1970.
49. Bailey, G.L.: Uremia as a total body disease, in Bailey, G.L. (ed): Hemodialysis Principles and Practice. New York, Academic Press Inc 1971, p 1.
50. Fredrickson, D.S., Levy, R.I., Lees, R.S.: Fat transport in lipopro- teins. An integrated approach to mechanisms and disorders. N Engl J Med 276:34, 1967.
51. Blankenhorn, D., Chin, H., Lau, F.: Ischemic heart disease in young adults. Metabolic and angiographic diagnosis and the prevalence of Type IV hyperlipoproteinemia. Ann Intern Med 69:21, 1968.
52. Burton, B.T., Krueger, K.K., Bryan, F.A.: National registry of long- term dialysis patients. JAMA 218:718, 1971.
53. Ninth report of the human renal transplantation registry, advisory com- mittee to the renal transplantation registry, JAMA 220:253, 1972.
54. Parsons, F.M., Brunner, F.P., Gurland, H.J., et al: Combined report on regular dialysis and transplantation in europe, I.: Proc Europ Dial Trans Assoc 8:3, 1971.
55. Lowrie, E.G., Lazarus, J.M., Mocelin, A.J., et al: A study of survivor- ship in patients undergoing chronic hemodialysis and renal trans- plantation. N Engl J Med. 288:863, 1973.
56. Bagdade, J., Porte D., Bierman, E.: Diabetic lipemia: a form of acquired fat-induced lipemia. N Engl J Med 276:427, 1967.
57. Reaven, G., Lerner, R., Stern, M., et al: Role of insulin in endogenous hypertriglyceridemia. J Clin Invest 46:1756, 1967.
58. Hubner, W., Siebert, H.G., Diemer, A., et al: Effects of regular haemo- dialysis with glucose and glucose-free dialysate on hyperlipaemia. Proc Europ Dial Trans Assoc 8:176, 1971.
59. Borst J.: Protein katabolism in uremia. Effects of protein free diet, in- fections, and blood transfusions. Lancet 1:824, 1948.
60. Shaw, A., Bazzard, F., Booth, E., et al: Treatment of chronic renal failure by a modified Giovannetti diet. Q J Med 34:237, 1965.
61. Giovannetti, S., Balestri, P., Biagini, M., et al: Implications of dietary therapy. Arch Intern Med 7:900, 1970.
62. Farr, L., Smadel, J.: The effect of dietary protein on the cause of nephro- toxic nephritis in rats. J Exp Med 70:615, 1939.
63. Rose, W.C., Dekker, E.E.: Urea as a source of nitrogen for the biosyn- thesis of amino acids. J Biol Chem 223:107, 1956.
64. Josephson, B., Bergstrom, J., Furst, P., et al: Studies on metabolism of urea, amino acids and protein in uremia patients, in Kluthe, R., Berlyne, G., Burton, B. (eds): Uremia. Stuttgart, Georg Thieme Verlag, 1972, p144.
65. Giordano, C., DeSanto, N., Rinaldi, S., et al: Histadine and glycine essential amino acids in uremia, in Kluthe, R., Berlyne, G., Burton, B. (eds): Uremia. Stuttgart, Georg Thieme Verlag, 1972, p 138.
66. Shear, L.: Internal redistribution of tissue protein synthesis in uremia. J Clin Invest 48:1252, 1969.

67. Giordano, C.: Use of exogenous and endogenous urea for protein synthesis in normal and uremic subjects. J Lab Clin Med 62:231, 1963.
68. Giordano, C., de Pascale, C., DeSanto, N., et al: Use of different sources of nitrogen in uremia. Arch Intern Med 126:787, 1970.
69. Giovannetti, S., Maggiore, Q.: A low nitrogen diet with proteins of high biological value for severe chronic uremia. Lancet 1:1000, 1964.
70. Berlyne, G., Shaw, A., Nilwarangkur, S.: Dietary treatment of chronic renal failure: Experience with a modified Giovannetti diet. Nephron 2:129, 1965.
71. Franklin, S., Gordon, A., Kleeman, C., et al: Use of a balanced low-protein diet in chronic renal failure. JAMA 202:477, 1967.
72. Berlyne, G., Shaw, A.: Giordano-Giovannetti diet in terminal renal failure. Lancet 2:7, 1967.
73. Kopple, J., Shinaberger, J., Coburn, J., et al: Evaluating modified protein diets for uremia. J Am Diet Assn 54:481, 1969.
74. Kopple, J., Shinaberger, J., Rubini, M., et al: Metabolic studies during protein restriction in uremic man. Clin Res 19:152, 1971.
75. Kopple, J., Shinaberger, J., Coburn, J., et al: Optimal dietary protein treatment during chronic hemodialysis. Trans Am Soc Artif Intern Organs 15:302, 1969.
76. Kopple, J., Coburn, J., Rubini, M.: Nitrogen requirements in uremia, in Kluthe, R., Berlyne, G., Burton, B. (eds): Uremia. Stuttgart, Georg Thieme Verlag, 1972, p 271.
77. Ginn, E., Frost, A., Lacy, W.: Nitrogen balance in hemodialysis patients. Am J Clin Nutr 21:385, 1968.
78. Bianchi, R., Mariani, G., Pilo, A.: Albumin metabolism in uremic patients on low protein diet, in Kluthe, R., Berlyne, G., Burton, B. (eds): Uremia. Stuttgart, Georg Thieme Verlag, 1972, p 206.
79. Bischel, M., Sabin, N., Homola, B., et al: Albumin turnover in chronically hemodialyzed patients. Trans Am Soc Artif Intern Organs 15:298, 1969.
80. Fish, J.C., Remmers, A., Jr., Lindley, J., et al: Albumin kinetics and and nutritional rehabilitation in the unattended home-dialysis patient. N Engl J Med 287:478, 1972.
81. Gulyassy, P.F., Peters, J.H., Lin, S.C., et al: Hemodialysis and plasma amino acid composition in chronic renal failure. Am J Clin Nutr 21:565, 1968.
82. Peters, J.H., Gulyassy, P., Lin, S., et al: Amino acid patterns in uremia: Comparative effects of hemodialysis and transplantation. Trans Am Soc Artif Intern Organs 14:405, 1968.
83. Gulyassy, P., Aviram, A., Peters, J.: Evaluation of amino acid and protein requirements in uremia. Arch Intern Med 126:855, 1970.
84. Meeting, D., Deshuk, B.: Free amino acids in serum, cerebrospinal fluid and urine in renal disease with and without uremia. Proc Exp Biol Med 126:754, 1967.
85. McMenamy, R., Oncley, J.: The specific binding of L-tryptophan to serum albumin. J Biol Chem 233:1436, 1956.

86. Gulyassy, P., Peters, J., Schoenfeld, P.: Transport and protein binding of tryptophan in uremia, in Kluthe, R., Berlyne, G., Burton, B. (eds): Uremia. Stuttgart, Georg Thieme Verlag, 1972, p 163.

87. Letteri, J.M., Melik, H., Louis, S., et al: Diphenylhydantoin metabolism in uremia. N Engl J Med 285:648, 1971.

88. Kopple, J., Wang, M., Vyhmeister, I., et al: Tyrosine metabolism in uremia, in Kluthe, R., Berlyne, G., Burton, B., (eds): Uremia. Stuttgart, Georg Thieme Verlag, 1972, p 150.

89. Taurian, A., Goddard, J., and Puck, T.: Phenylalanine hydroxylase activity in mammalian cells. J Cell Physiol 73:159, 1969.

90. Wong, R.G., Norman, A.W., Reddy, C.R., et al: Biologic effects of 1,25-dihydroxycholecalciferol (a highly active vitamin D metabolite) in acutely uremic rats. J Clin Invest 51:1287, 1972.

91. Beckers, C., van Ypersela de Strihou, C., Coche, E., et al: Iodine metabolism in severe renal insufficiency. J Clin Endocrinol Metab 29:293, 1969.

92. Ramirez, G., Jubiz, W., Gutch, C., et al: Thyroid function in chronic renal failure: Effects of chronic hemodialysis. Trans Am Soc Artif Intern Organs 18:224, 1972.

93. Ibid. Discussion of manuscript, p 248.

94. Elstein, M., Smith, E., Curtis, J.: Reproductive potential of patients treated by maintenance hemodialysis. Br Med J 2:734, 1969.

95. Confortini, P., Galanti, G., Ancona, G., et al: Full-term pregnancy and successful delivery in a patient on chronic hemodialysis. Proc Europ Dial Trans Assoc 8:74, 1971.

96. Ibid. Discussion of manuscript, p 78.

97. Lindsay, R., Briggs, J., Luke, R., et al: Gynaecomastia in chronic renal failure. Br Med J 4:779, 1967.

98. Freeman, R., Lawton, R., Fearing, N.: Gynecomastia: An endocrinologic complication of hemodialysis. Ann Intern Med 69:67, 1968.

99. Schmidt, G., Shehadeah, I., Swain, C.: Transient gynecomastia in chronic renal failure during chronic intermittent hemodialysis. Ann Intern Med 78:73, 1968.

10
The Skeletal System

Although for many years uremia has been known to be associated with abnormal calcium metabolism [1,2], the severity and extent of the defect has been appreciated only since the introduction of chronic hemodialysis and renal transplantation [3,4]. By prolonging the life of patients with chronic renal failure, these procedures have resulted in an exaggeration of bone pathology (with clinical implications), and heretofore have not been fully emphasized. (Figure 1.)

There seems little doubt that defective absorption of calcium from the gut is one of the prime factors resulting in abnormal calcium metabolism in chronic renal failure [2]. A physiological resistance to large doses of vitamin D was reported in 1943 by Liu and Chu [2]. These investigators also commented on the skeletal lesions in their patients which they noted were similar to those seen in rickets or simple osteomalacia. While vitamin D resistance has been confirmed by others [5,6], its exact pathophysiological mechanism—although recently clarified considerably—remains somewhat obscured, as exemplified by data showing normal intestinal absorption of calcium with enhanced, endogenous intestinal secretion in patients with chronic renal failure [7].

The main circulating form of vitamin D_3 is 25-hydroxycholecalciferol (25-HCC) [8], and this is produced by hydroxylation in the liver from the parent substance. When the plasma calcium is low, 25-HCC is further metabolized in the kidneys to 1,25-dihydroxycholecalciferol (1,25-DHCC); when the plasma calcium is high, it is metabolized

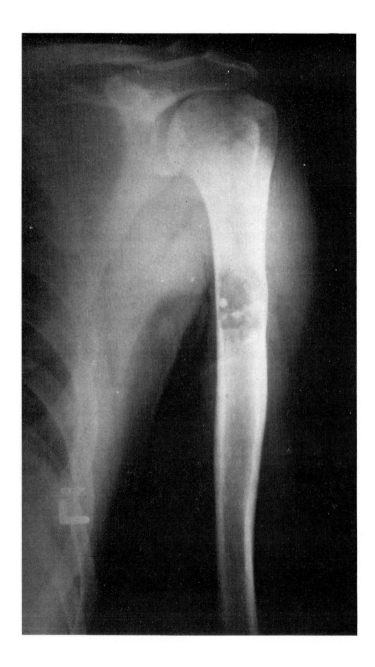

Fig. 1. Severe secondary hyperparathyroidism in individual entering a dialysis program. Note distal clavicle resorption and Brown tumor in upper humerus.

to 21,25-dihydroxycholecalciferol. The 1,25 derivative is the most active form of the vitamin so far discovered. After production by the kidneys, it is taken up by the intestines and bones [9,10]. Therefore, the kidneys may be regarded as endocrine organs producing a calcium-regulating hormone at a rate dependent upon the serum calcium level. Alterations in the metabolism of vitamin D or its hydroxylated metabolites in uremia may result in an accumulation of structurally related abnormal metabolites which compete with 1,25-DHCC for receptor sites in specific target organs. The end result in the bone is a decreased or defective mineralization of collagen, probably secondary to a maturation arrest of the collagen tissue.

Galante and his collegues [11] have demonstrated that parathyroid extract and, therefore, probably parathyroid hormone suppress the conversion of 25-HCC to 1,25-DHCC and enhance the conversion to 21,25-DHCC. Their data suggest that this is due to direct action of the hormone on the kidneys, although the authors are cautious to point out that other possible explanations are available. This raises the possibility that the severity of bone disease found in patients with renal failure may be due in part to the interference with vitamin D metabolism produced by high circulating levels of parathyroid hormone. Thus, some of the benefits which follow parathyroidectomy may be due to a removal of this block in vitamin D metabolism.

This phenomenon of vitamin D resistance has been attributed to uremic toxins interfering with normal conversion of vitamin D to its more active metabolites and/or altered response of the end organ to these metabolites. Recent studies with radioisotopic forms of vitamin D_3 and 25-HCC in subjects with renal failure [12,13], in anephric animals [14,15], and in animals with experimentally induced chronic renal failure [16] have focused attention on the loss of kidney *cells* rather than on the loss of *excretory* function as being responsible for the defect in intestinal calcium transport. One would anticipate that a reduction in kidney mass would result in a decreased renal production of 1,25-DHCC. It is likely that the subsequent reduction in the intestinal mucosal concentration of 1,25-DHCC leads to a progressive decrease in calcium absorption. Results demonstrating that small doses of 1,25-DHCC increase calcium absorption and the level of serum calcium of uremic man are consistent with this hypothesis [17].

Moreover, many patients with chronic renal failure may be treated with diphenylhydantoin and phenobarbitol. Recent studies [18] show that this combination of anticonvulsant drugs may result in low levels of 25-HCC in *nonuremic* man, and these findings may be extrapolated to the uremic patient. These drugs, therefore, may compound an already deranged vitamin D metabolism in uremic patients.

Alterations in the metabolic fate of 25-HCC do not as yet completely explain the calcium malabsorption of uremia. Defects in calcium absorption are noted in renal insufficiency at a time when the metabolism of vitamin D and the tissue localization of metabolites are said to be normal [19]. Some data, however, indicate that vitamin D therapy alone reverses the osteomalacia of bilaterally nephrectomized patients on hemodialysis [29] and that 25-HCC is effective therapy for patients with uremic bone disease and individuals refractory to equivalent doses of vitamin D [21]. As indicated previously, these latter findings suggest that in end-stage renal failure refractoriness to vitamin D may involve end-organ failure secondary to a variety of uremic circulating factors as well as defective vitamin D metabolism.

Bricker and associates [22,23] have postulated that secondary hyperparathyroidism in chronic renal failure begins with the first phase of nephron destruction and progresses in severity with progressive nephron loss. They postulate that in order to maintain phosphate homeostasis as glomerular filtration rate decreases, greater phosphate-losing capacity is required from individual nephrons. Transient increases in serum phosphate reciprocally decrease serum calcium, which proceeds to stimulate parathyroid hormone. The end result of the increased hormone level is that phosphate excretion in the tubule is enhanced and phosphate balance is restored. Obviously nephron destruction progresses to phosphate imbalance, and hyperphosphatemia results. These investigators postulate that careful control of phosphate intake in the early phases of renal failure may alleviate or *prevent* the development of secondary hyperparathyroidism [24].

Chronic renal failure with its accompanying hyperphosphatemia and hypocalcemia leads to progressive hyperplasia and hypertrophy of parathyroid glands. The glands may enlarge markedly and some data indicate that this roughly correlates with the degree of bone disease and the level of parathyroid hormone in the serum [25].

Conversely, evidence also indicates that functional hyperparathyroidism may occur in a mattter of weeks following the onset of uremia. The occurrence of hypercalcemia in the diuretic phase of acute renal failure appears to bear this out [26], as do more recent experiments showing an elevated parathyroid hormone level in patients with acute renal failure [27].

The responsiveness of the uremic parathyroid gland to changes in serum calcium concentration has not been well defined, but is probably variable. In response to persistent long-standing hypocalcemia, the enlarged hyperplastic tissue may become insensitive to the usual factors that regulate secretion. This may result in a state of autonomy which produces *hyper*calcemia when uremia is corrected by techniques such as dialysis or transplantation [28]. From our experience, it seems that this autonomy is not an "all or none" affair. This is emphasized by the observation that some patients may develop mild *hyper*calcemia and intensification of bone lesions following successful renal homotransplantation [29]. If left to their own resources, these individuals most often return to a euparathyroid level after 6 to 12 months [30]. Prolonged hypercalcemia not suppressible by oral drug therapy (e.g., oral phosphate) continues in another group of patients and results in progressive bone disease. This latter phenomenon is becoming more common in our experience and may be in some way related to aseptic necrosis of the joinits in the post-transplant period [31].

The role of acidosis in the development of uremic osteodystrophy is not known. From the observation of Goodman and co-workers [32], it is likely that the skeleton acts as a buffer of excess hydrogen ion in chronic renal failure. Although no direct available evidence indicates that acidosis can activate a mechanism for resorption of whole bone in the sense that parathyroid hormone does, it is nevertheless possible that acidosis produces bone demineralization while utilizing calcium phosphate as a buffer [33].

Uremia usually causes a decrease in the serum calcium level, which—in rare instances and when the acidosis is mild or when sodium bicarbonate is administered with a resultant rapid correction of acidosis—results in frank tetany. Serum phosphate also increases and may be followed by an elevated serum alkaline phosphatase activity. The latter, in our experience, correlates roughly with the severity of bone involvement. Osteodystrophy accompanying chronic renal failure depends on many factors. It seems logical that if the skeleton is capable of responding to an excess of parathyroid hormone through whatever interrelationships it may have with vitamin D metabolism, osteitis fibrosa cystica will be the predominant bone pathology. Under these circumstances, the [Ca] × [P] product is usually abnormally high, and this may lead to ectopic calcification in soft tissues. This phenomenon is not rare in uremic and quite common in dialysis patients who are either not restricting phosphate intake or not taking oral phosphate binders. It may be seen in the eyes as band keratopathy or conjunctivitis secondary to calcium deposits in the conjunctiva; in or around the joints as large ectopic soft tissue masses or frank arthritis resembling gouty arthritis; in the blood vessels as calcification of the medial layer; and in the skin calcium deposits may be associated with severe pruritus, especially in patients on maintenance dialysis [34,35]. Furthermore, Berlyne and co-workers [36] suggest that cataracts result from prolonged hypocalcemia as a result of chronic renal failure, and, although we have no hard data to substantiate it, our clinical impression is that cataracts are more common in this population. Severe metastatic calcifications around blood vessels may result in ischemic ulcerations of skin and necrosis of muscle as pointed out by Richardson and associates [37].

When the primary physiologic lesion is secondary to vitamin D resistance or deficiency, osteomalacia rather than osteitis fibrosa cystica is the predominant lesion [38]. Under these conditions, the serum calcium concentration may be somewhat lower than one might expect to find in the face of a given phosphate concentration. Moreover, x-rays and bone biopsies show that the majority of patients have areas of osteitis fibrosa cystica and osteomalacia, in addition to osteosclerosis and diffuse osteoporosis. (Figure 2.)

Although 25-HCC or 1,25-DHCC may prove to be effective therapeutic agents, the supply of 25-HCC is quite limited and the sythesis of 1,25-DHCC is presently too expensive to make it routinely available [19]. And, as pointed out by Avioli [19], both may be inappropriate therapeutic agents in chronic renal failure since their ability to activate intestinal calcium absorption is probably accompanied by an exaggeration of bone resorption. Avioli further points out that it is likely that the reported hypercalcemic-hypophosphatemic response of uremic patients to limited 1,25-DHCC therapy may reflect a combination of stimulated intestinal calcium transport and skeletal osteolysis. Therefore, further information about these substances is required before their biological effectiveness in uremic man can be clearly predicted. Despite these reservations, however, Brickman and associates [39] have demonstrated that 1,25-DHCC effectively increases intestinal calcium absorption in a small group of uremic patients. Further clinical trials will most certainly follow.

The role of magnesium in the osteodystrophy of renal failure is obscure and, to date, its contribution has been largely ignored in most therapeutic programs. Serum magnesium concentrations in patients with chronic renal failure maintained by dialysis are not generally markedly elevated unless large amounts of magnesium containing antacids for phosphate binding are ingested. It is of interest, however, that renal excretion of magnesium in contrast to calcium continues in significant amounts despite severe renal failure [38]. Furthermore, there is clear evidence that magnesium influences the secretion of parathyroid hormone both in vivo [40] and in vitro [41]. The theoretical suppression of parathyroid hormone by means of hypermagnesemia may have practical implications in the dialysis situation. Pletka et al [42] have presented

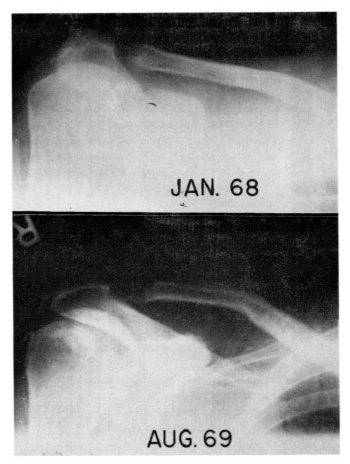

Fig. 2. Progression of osteitis fibrosa cystica in patient being maintained with the artificial kidney. There is clear evidence of progression of distal resorption of clavicle after 18 months of treatment.

preliminary information indicating that significant suppression of the parathyroid gland is possible by dialyzing patients against a slightly increased magnesium concentration. By keeping the dialysate-magnesium concentration at 2.6 mEq/L, he demonstrated a significant drop in parathyroid hormone levels over a 6-month period.

It is also of interest that *hypo*magnesemia may interfere with calcium release from bone with resultant hypocalcemia. This relationship should be considered in the patient with chronic renal failure. Repletion of magnesium stores under these circumstances improves the serum calcium level. Despite this, however, Kleeman and co-workers [38] were unable to demonstrate any specific inter-relationship between total and diffusible plasma magnesium and calcium.

The role of calcitonin in the deranged calcium metabolism of renal failure is unknown. The exact function of this hormone is also unclear, but is likely that along with parathyroid hormone it has a significant role in regulating blood calcium levels. This regulation may be achieved jointly by parathyroid hormone and calcitonin, i.e., oscillations in blood calcium produced by changes in the secretion rate of parathyroid hormone, the slower acting hormone, are prevented by calcitonin. In addition, calcitonin may moderate bone growth and remodeling and, by preventing the action of parathyroid hormone on bone, calcitonin may allow the calcium-conserving effect of the kidneys and gut to remain unopposed [43].

The vast majority of patients with severe renal failure and almost all individuals who have been maintained by the artificial kidney for a long period of time show some histologic evidence of parathyroid hyperplasia and x-ray evidence of early bone resorption. Fortunately, only a small percentage of these patients develop clinical abnormalities of bone metabolism which requires specific treatment. In our experience, approximately 10 percent of the patients entering a dialysis-transplantation program manifest evidence of *severe* clinical renal osteodystrophy [25].

While it has been helpful *clinically* to divide renal osteodystrophy into two categories—osteomalacia and osteitis fibrosa cystica—pathologic examination of bone in uremia usually shows a mixture of lesions as outlined above.

The treatment of the uremic patient with marked parathyroid hyperfunction (osteitis fibrosa cystica) is difficult not only because of the problems of recognizing pure forms of the disorder but because treatment of one abnormality often results in the aggravation of another. The task of treating these patients has not been made easier by long-term dialysis which, by prolonging the life of the terminal uremic patient, has also made possible the expression of a more severe form of the disease.

When the major bone pathology or x-ray examination indicates osteomalacia and especially when this is accompanied by marked hypocalcemia, the use of some form of vitamin D and/or calcium supplement is a rational therapeutic approach. Since dihydrotachysterol (DHT) activity is not reduced by absence of the kidneys [44] whereas activities of other forms of vitamin D probably are, there is some theoretical reason for using this steroid in patients with chronic renal failure. We have had some experience with this method and have found it quite effective. One must be cautious in using DHT, however, since *hyper*calcemia commonly results. This form of therapy has a beneficial long-term effect in some patients and in animals [45-48]. Nevertheless, the interplay of parathyroid hypertrophy (and an increased level of parathyroid hormone) which is not totally responsive to mechanisms normally controlling parathyroid secretion [49] should be kept in mind when administering vitamin D or its derivatives. Serum calcium level should be carefully monitored during the administration of the vitamin, since treatment with calcium and high doses of vitamin D in any form sometimes leads to hypercalcemia and, if the [Ca] × [P] product is elevated sufficiently, to the ectopic precipitation of calcium salts [50,51]. (Figure 3.)

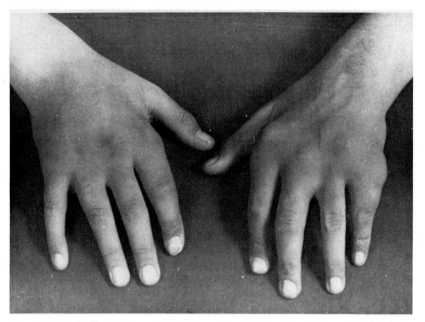

Fig. 3. Marked ectopic calcifications surrounding hand joints in individual entering a dialysis program.

As pointed out by Bailey and associates [52], avascular necrosis of the joints may occur in a dialysis population. Although these patients do not commonly show symptomatic involvement of the joints, they do show x-ray evidence of this phenomenon. The cause is obscure, but hyperparathyroidism is believed to be the primary event. Perhaps exposure of hyperparathyroid lesion to large doses of corticosteroids in the post-transplant period result in a high incidence of symptomatic aseptic necrosis.

As a general guideline to the therapeutic assessment of the effects of vitamin D and supplemental calcium for the treatment of osteomalacic renal osteodystrophy, one should measure the serum calcium level frequently and reduce or discontinue treatment when calcium rises to the normal range or the alkaline phosphatase level returns to normal. The effect of high doses of vitamin D may persist for some time [47]. Patients who have bone disease manifest by bone pain may show significant improvement in these symptoms following several weeks of vitamin D and calcium therapy, while a radiographic and histologic changes become evident only after a more prolonged period of time.

The use of phosphate binders to depress the serum phosphate level and thereby reciprocally lower parathyroid hormone (by increasing serum calcium) has theoretical merit [53]. We feel its use in long-term dialysis patients is mandatory, and we have seen ectopic calcifications come and go depending on how fastidiously patients ingest these antacids [54]. Others have also documented this [53], and, whenever possible, we use *nonmagnesium*-containing anatacids in individuals undergoing chronic dialysis. Periodic checks of serum phosphorus are required to adjust the dose of the phosphate binders. Occasionally, constipation is a consequence of excess ingestion of these substances and the type of antacid used must be individualized. The potentially hazardous problems with constipation was discussed in Chapter 7. (Figure 4.)

Management of the patient with persistent "high normal" or frankly elevated serum calcium values requires a different therapeutic approach. When there is also radiographic evidence of osteitis fibrosa cystica and/or considerably ectopic calcification in soft tissues unresponsive to phosphate control, parathyroidectomy is the preferred treatment [25,55]. Patients with frank hypercalcemia are thought to have developed a form of "autonomous" hyperparathyroidism and conservative treatment, in our experience, has been uniformly unsuccessful. Subtotal parathyroidectomy (removing 3-½ glands) [56] or total parathyroidectomy [57] does not result in a severe postoperative morbidity or mortality and alleviates hypercalcemia [56].

We have found that parathyroid hyperplasia is not limited to patients with osteitis fibrosa cystica, but is also found in most patients with roentgenographic of histologic evidence of osteomalacia [25] as the primary lesion. Chief-cell hyperplasia or a combination of chief- and clear-cell hyperplasia were found in the parathyroid glands of all patients who had predominant osteomalacic lesions and in the vast majority of patients with diffuse skeletal demineralization not diagnostic of osteomalacia. Two other patients whose glands were not examined

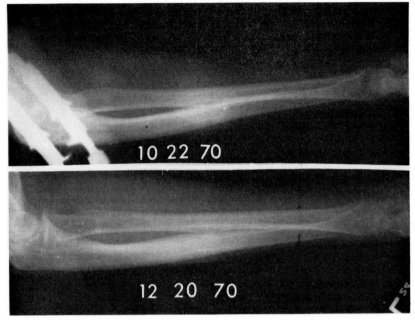

Fig. 4. Marked decrease in soft tissue calcification following institution of phosphate-lowering (antacid) therapy. Individual had been treated with hemodialysis for 4 years and developed lesions following interruption of antacid therapy. Deposits are almost totally resorbed after only 2 months of serum phosphate control.

had markedly elevated circulating parathyroid levels. These findings indicate the complexity of the clinical picture and the potential hazards of one form of treatment versus another. Since parathyroid hyperfunction is invariably present in renal osteodystrophy—regardless of the type of bone disease—and vitamin D and calcium therapy are not without risk and may be contraindicted in some patients, surgical removal of the hyperplastic parathyroid tissue is the logical therapeutic approach when there is some doubt as to the "form" of osteodystrophy present. Appropriate vitamin D and calcium therapy may follow surgical removal.

Of course, not all patients undergoing chronic dialysis require parathyroidectomy. Our criterion for selection is that the patient has some form of symptomatic bone disease, and indications for surgery include progression of roentgenographic evidence of bone disease, frank hypercalcemia, and ectopic calcifications such as progressive medial vascular calcification unresponsive to therapy. The last phenomenon,

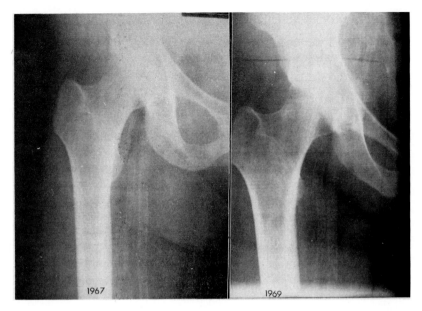

Fig. 5. Vascular calcifications that have remained essentially unchanged 2 years after successful renal homotransplantation. In 1969, patient's serum creatinine was approximately 1.0 mg/100 ml and all other evidence of secondary hyperparathyroidism had disappeared.

quite common in patients undergoing chronic hemodialysis, is very difficult if not impossible to reverse. Since vascular compromise can result from progressive vascular calcification, we consider this an indication for early therapy. (Figure 5.)

There is some evidence which is growing in scope [58] that the dialysate-calcium concentration can affect the progression of renal osteodystrophy. It now seems apparent that maintenance of calcium levels to between 6 and 7 mg/100 ml in the dialysate may be beneficial. Some studies [59,60] show objective evidence of healing of bone disease under these circumstances. In a preliminary study [61], we found that 5 mg/100 ml maintained over many months was insufficient to produce a lowering in parathyroid hormone levels. However, 6.5 mg/100 ml appears to be effective and needs further study over longer periods. Again, serum phosphate concentration must be carefully controlled, as there may be interdialysis or immediate postdialysis transient hypercalcemia and the [Ca] × [P] product must be monitored. As indicated earlier, evidence also suggests that an increase in the magnesium concentration of the dialysis bath is beneficial [42].

Our experience indicates that over many months or years, serum parathyroid hormone concentration tends to increase in the majority of patients being maintained with the artificial kidney; therefore, any indication that the progression of osteodystrophy is arrested or improved is important. Since only a small group of patients have symptomatic bone disease when entering a dialysis program, the ability to contain it (if not the ability to improve it) by any therapeutic modality is worthy of trail. Nevertheless, we have rarely seen *severe* bone disease improve spontaneously during dialysis, and in less than a handful of patients can we clearly document such improvement. (Figure 6.)

Although some individuals have suggested that total parathyroidectomy [57] is the treatment of choice for secondary hyperparathyroidism when surgery is contemplated, we use a subtotal surgical approach. Since most patients in our dialysis program are potential candidates for renal homotransplantation, we feel that leaving behind a small amount of parathyroid tissue decreases surgical morbidity and maintains a normal mineral metabolism once a well-functioning allograft is present. Although in time the *re*currence of secondary hyperparathyroidism is to be expected we have had to reoperate in only 2 of 75 cases of subtotal parathyroidectomy. (Figure 7.)

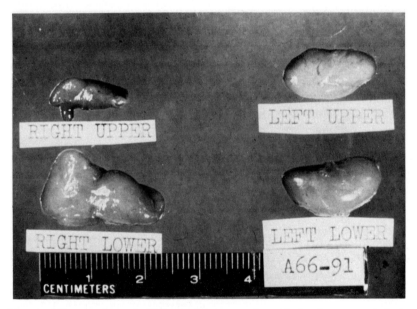

Fig. 6.   Three and one-half hyperplastic parathyroid glands removed during surgery.

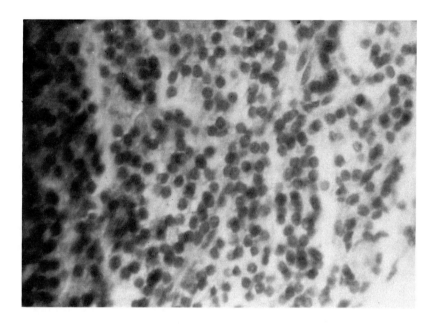

Fig. 7. Histological specimen taken at surgical removal of parathyroid glands. Note marked chief cell hyperplasia.

Subtotal parathyroidectomy involves removing all identifiable parathyroid glands except one-half of the smallest gland, leaving behind less than one-eighth of the original parathyroid tissue. There has been no operative mortality in our series, and symptoms are usually limited to moderate pain at the incision site for 24 to 48 hours. Most individuals return home within 5 days of surgery.

Serum calcium falls within 48 hours of surgery in all patients and generally returns to normal in those who are severely hypercalcemic. Subsequently, it may decrease, occasionally to levels as low as 3.5 mg/100 ml. Patients operated on and maintained with regular dialysis are generally entirely asymptomatic, whereas nondialyzed patients may show mild tetany and require temporary calcium and vitamin D therapy.

This course is extremely variable, however, and many exceptions occur. After 2 weeks to 1 month, serum calcium usually levels off, regardless of whether or not patients are treated with some form of vitamin D and calcium, and subsequently gradually rises to the normal or low-normal range. Patients who exhibit severe hypocalcemia with symptoms in the immediate postoperative period may require prolonged therapy but this is variable. Following parathyroidectomy, alkaline phosphatase level either remains elevated or rises even further for several weeks [25,56].

Other than correction of hypercalcemia, the most striking feature of parathyroidectomy is the rapid resorption of soft tissue calcium deposits. Both subcutaneous and periarticular calcification may decrease considerably within the first few weeks and tend to disappear within the first few months of surgery. By contrast and of significant importance is the fact that in our experience, contrary to that of others [62], none of the vascular calcifications disappear completely and most of them remain totally unchanged.

Bone pain usually disappears shortly after surgery and bone repair is detectible in serial x-rays within a few weeks to a few months. As might be expected, the rate of remineralization and the time required for its completion correlates roughly with the degree of preexisting bone loss, although individual variations are common. (Figure 8.)

An unexpected finding following subtotal parathyroidectomy in patients being maintained with the artificial kidney was the disappearance of pruritus [34,35]. This may be related to surgical removal of ectopic calcium salt deposits in the skin [34]. We have also seen a patient who complained of severe uncontrollable pruritus without other evidence of hyperparathyroid overactivity. His bone x-rays were normal and serum calcium levels were not elevated. Immediately after parathyroidectomy, the itching disappeared.

Because of this initial favorable experience, we recently performed subtotal parathyroidectomy on 3 other patients who complained of itching but showed no other evidence of bone disease. The itching disappeared in 1 individual, and was unaffected in the other 2. These cases illustrate the mistake of indiscriminate use of subtotal parathyroidectomy to "cure" pruritus. Unfortunately, we know of no way to predict which individuals (without bone disease) will respond to subtotal parathyroidectomy and which will not. In our present state of the art, we would *not* recommend parathyroidectomy for pruritus in the absence of clear indications of metabolic bone disease.

The role of fluoride in treating or aggravating renal osteodystrophy remains to be elucidated. Some data had suggested that it was extremely

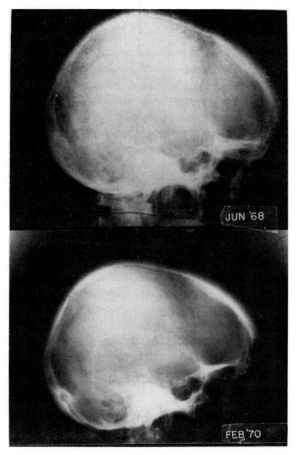

Fig. 8. Marked improvement in secondary skull hyper-parathyroidism in patient maintained with artificial kidney for approximately 18 months. In our experience such improvement is unusual without parathyroidectomy.

detrimental to chronic dialysis patients [63]. We believe that these data are preliminary at best and that the information presented does not justify such a conclusion. We have had several patients who have undergone dialysis in areas where the water has been fluoridated, and bone disease has not progressed rapidly in these patients. One patient was dialyzed for 5 years with fluoridated water. We currently use water purification methods whenever possible on simply theoretical grounds, but do not institute such purification methods solely for the removal of fluoride. Our clinical impression is that *if* fluoride is detrimental at all, its effects are not seen for some time. Certainly, no evidence to date indicates that *drinking* fluoridated water has any detrimental effect on patients with renal failure [64].

Muscle cramps, a common occurrence in patients with uremia [65], can be a bothersome clinical problem. They are most common at night but may occur anytime. Patients treated with artificial kidneys may also experience muscle cramps. In most instances, the cramps occur late in the course of dialysis, and are due to or precipitated by dehydration. The judicious use of saline during these episodes generally effectively controls them. Cramps may preceed clinical hypotension by some time, and can be a useful clinical tool in medical management.

Other patients experience cramps between or during dialysis that do not appear to be directly related to fluid balance. What role calcium, magnesium, and/or changes in pH (alkalosis with dialysis) play in these cramps is speculative. When dialyzing patients (for experimental purposes) against a low-calcium dialysate, we have found that cramps are common. Furthermore, we have found that during the first few dialyses with an elevated magnesium dialysate (i.e., 2.6 mEq/L), cramps are also quite common but subside with time even though dialysate magnesium remains constant.

We have found that in some patients quinine alone effectively controls cramps between dialyses. Conversely, in other patients quinine is totally ineffective and some other method of control is required. Occasionally patients can be "cured" simply by elevating the calcium content in the dialysate. Others respond to a change in dialysate-magnesium concentration, and still others are unaffected by either maneuver. Sometimes cramps are severe enough to require narcotics during the dialysis procedure. We stress, however, that this is quite unusual and generally one of the above methods for controlling cramps is effective.

REFERENCES

1. Schreiner, G.E., Maher, J.F.: Uremia: Biochemistry and pathogenesis—Treatment. New York, C.C. Thomas, 1961.
2. Liu, S.A., Chu,H.I.: Studies of calcium and phosphorus metabolism with special reference to the pathogenesis and effect of dehydratochysterol, (AT 10) and iron. Medicine (Baltimore) 22:103, 1943.
3. Hampers, C.L., Schupak, E.: Long-Term Hemodialysis: Management of the patient with chronic renal failure. New York, Grune & Stratton, 1967.

4. Pendras, J.P., Erickson, R.V.: Hemodialysis: A successful therapy for chronic uremia. Ann Intern Med 64:293, 1966.
5. Dent, C.E., Harper, C.M., Philpot, G.R.: The treatment of renal glomerular osteodystrophy. Q J Med 30:1, 1961.
6. Stanbury, S.W., Lumb, G.A.: Metabolic studies of renal osteodystrophy: I. Calcium, phosphorus and nitrogen metabolism in rickets, osteomalacia and hyperparathyroidism complicating chronic uremia. Medicine (Baltimore) 41:1, 1962.
7. Gonick, H.C., Hertoghe, J., Rubini, M.E.: Disorders of calcium metabolism in uremia. (abstract) J Clin Invest 44:1053, 1965.
8. Blunt, J.W., DeLuca, H.F., Schnoes, H.D.: 25-Hydroxycholecalciferol. A biological active metabolite of vitamin D. Biochemistry 7:3317, 1968.
9. Myrtle, J.F., Norman, A.W.: Vitamin D—A cholecalciferol metabolite highly active in promoting intestinal calcium transport. Science 171: 79, 1971.
10. Haussler, M.R., Boyce, D.W., Littledike, E.T., et al: A rapidly acting metabolite of vitamin D . Proc Natl Acad Sci USA 68:177, 1971.
11. Galante, L., MacAuley, S., Colston, K., et al: Effect of parathyroid extract vitamin D metabolism. Lancet 1:985, 1972.
12. Mawer, E.B., Backhouse, J., Lumb, G.A., et al: Evidence for formation of 1,25-dihydroxycholecalciferol during metabolism of vitamin D in man. Nature 232:188, 1971.
13. Avioli, L.V., Birge, S.J., Lee, S.E., et al: The metabolic fate of vitamin D_3-^3H in chronic renal failure. J Clin Invest 47:2239, 1968.
14. Gray, R., Boyle, I., DeLuca, H.F.: Vitamin D metabolism: The role of kidney tissue. Science 172:1232, 1971.
15. Hill, L.F., VanDenBerg, C.J., Mawer, E.B.:Vitamin D metabolism in experimental uremia: Effects on intestinal transport 45 Ca and on formation of 1,25-dihydroxycholecalciferol in rat. Nature 232:189, 1971.
16. Avioli, L.V., Birge, S.J., Slatopolsky, E.: The nature of vitamin D resistance of patients with chronic renal disease. Arch Intern Med 124: 451, 1969.
17. Brickman, A.S., Coburn, J.W., Norman, A.W.: Action of 1,25-dihydroxycholecalciferol, A potent kidney-produced metabolite of vitamin D_3 in uremic man. N Engl J Med 287:891, 1972.
18. Hahn, T.J., Hendin, B.A., Sharp, C.R., et al: Effect of chronic anticonvulsant therapy on serum 25-hydroxycalciferol levels in adults. N Engl J Med 287:900, 1972.
19. Avioli, L.V.: Vitamin D, the kidney and calcium hemeostasis. Kidney Internat 2:241, 1972.
20. Stanbury, S.W.: Azotemic renal osteodystrophy in MacIntyre, I, (ed): Clinic in Endocrinology Metabolism, vol 1. Philadelphia, W.B. Saunders Co., 1972, p 271.
21. Witmer, G., Balsan, S.: 25-hydroxycholecalciferol. Effects in renal osteodystrophy in working party on mineral metabolism. Éuropean Society for Pedriatric Research, 1971.
22. Bricker, N.S.: Invited discussion. Arch Intern Med 124:292, 1969.

23. Slatopolsky, E., Caglar, S., Gradowska, L., et al: On the prevention of secondary hyperparathyroidism in experimental chronic renal disease using "proportional reduction" of dietary phosphorus intake. Kidney Internat 2:147, 1972.
24. Slatopolsky, E., Rutherford, W.E., Hoffstein, P.E., Elkan, I.O., Butcher, H.E., and Bricker, N.S.: Non-suppressible secondary hyperparathyroidism in chronic progressive renal disease. Kidney Internat 1:38, 1972.
25. Katz, A.I., Hampers, C.L., Merrill, J.P.: Secondary hyperparathyroidism and renal osteodystrophy in chronic renal failure. Medicine (Baltimore) 48:333, 1969.
26. Segal, A.J., Miller, M., Moses, A.M.: Hypercalcemia during the diuretic phase of acute renal failure. Ann Int Med 68:1066, 1968.
27. Massry, S.G., Coburn, J.W., Glassock, R., et al: Divalent ion metabolism and renal osteodystrophy in chronic renal failure and effects of chronic hemodialysis and renal transplantation. Sixth Annual Contractor's Conference; Artificial Kidney-Chronic Uremia Program (Feb, 1973) p 26.
28. Katz, A.I., Hampers, C.L., Wilson, R.E., et al: The pace of subtotal parathyroidectomy in the management of patients with chronic renal failure. Trans Am Soc Artif Intern Organs 14:376, 1968.
29. McPhaul, J.U., Jr., McIntosh, D.S., Hammond, W.A., et al: Autonomous secondary (renal) parathyroid hyperplasia. N Engl J Med 271: 1342, 1964.
30. Hampers, C.L., Katz, A.I., Wilson, R.E., et al: Calcium metabolism and osteodystrophy after renal transplantation. Arch Intern Med 124: 282, 1969.
31. Briggs, W.A., Hampers, C.L., Merrill, J.P., et al: Aseptic necrosis in the femur after renal transplantation. Ann Surg 175:282, 1972.
32. Goodman, A.D., Lemann, J., Lennon, E.J., et al: Production excretion and net balance of fixed acid in patients with renal acidosis. J Clin Invest 44:495, 1965.
33. Stanbury, S.W.: Bone disease in uremia. Am J Med 44:714, 1968.
34. Massry, S.G., Popovtzer, M.M., Coburn, J.W., et al: Intractable pruritus as a manifestation of secondary hyperparathyroidism in uremia. N Engl J Med 279:697, 1968.
35. Hampers, C.L., Katz, A.I., Wilson, R.E., et al: Disappearance of "uremic" itching after subtotal parathyroidectomy. N Engl J Med 279: 695, 1968.
36. Berlyne, G.M., Ari, J.B., Danovitch, G.M., et al: Cataracts of chronic renal failure. Lancet 1:509, 1972. 4, 1972, p 509.
37. Richardson, J.A., Herron, G., Reitz, R., et al: Ischemic ulcerations of skin and necrosis of muscle in azotemic hyperparathyroidism. Ann Intern Med 71:129, 1969.
38. Kleeman, C.R., Better, O., Massry, S.G., et al: Divalent ion metabolism and osteodystrophy in chronic renal failure. Yale J Biol Med 40:1, 1967.

39. Brickman, A.S., Coburn, J.W., Norman, A.W.: Use of 1,25-dihydroxy-cholecalciferol in uremic man. N Engl J Med 287:891, 1972.
40. Gitelman, H.J., Kukolj, S., Welt, L.G.: The influence of the parathyroid glands on the hypercalcemia of experimental magnesium depletion in the rat. J Clin Invest 47:118, 1968.
41. Sherwood, L.M., Herrman, I., Bassett, C.A.: Parathyroid hormone secretion in vitro: Regulation by calcium and magnesium ions. Nature 25:1056, 1970.
42. Pletka, P., Bernstein, D.S., Hampers, C.L., et al: Effects of magnesium on parathyroid hormone secretion during chronic hemodialysis. Lancet 2:462, 1971.
43. Foster, G.W.: Calcitonin (Thyroicalcitonin). N Engl J Med 279:349, 1968.
44. Harrison, H.E., Harrison, H.C.: Dihydrotachysterol: A calcium active steroid not dependent upon kidney metabolism. J Clin Invest 51:1919, 1972.
45. Kaye, M.: Concepts of therapy. Arch Intern Med 124:656, 1969.
46. Hibberd, K.A., Norman, A.W.: Comparative biological effects of vitamin D_2 and D_3 and dihydrotachysterol$_2$ and dihydrotachysterol$_3$ in the chick. Biochem Pharmacol 18:2347, 1969.
47. Chen, P.S., Terepka, R.A., Overslaugh, C.: Hypercalcemia and hyperphosphotemic actions of dihydrotachysterol vitamin D_2 and hytakerd (AT 10) in rats and dogs. Endocrinology 70:815, 1962.
48. Kaye, M., Chatterjee, G., Cohen, G.F., et al: Arrest of hyperparathyroid bone disease with dihydrotachysterol in patients undergoing chronic hemodialysis. Ann Intern Med 73:225, 1970.
49. Popovtzer, M.M., Massey, S.G., Coburn, J.W., et al: Calcium infusion test in renal failure. (abstract) Proc. Third Annual Meeting Am Society of Nephrol, Dec, 1969.
50. Davidson, R.C., Pendras, J.P.: Calcium-related cardiorespiratory death in chronic hemodialysis. Trans Am Soc Artif Intern Organs 13:36, 1967.
51. Kim, D., Bell, N.H., Bundesen, W., et al: Renal osteodystrophy in the course of periodic dialysis for chronic uremia. Trans Am Soc Artif Intern Organs 14:367, 1968.
52. Bailey, G.L., Griffiths, H.J., Mocelin, A.J., et al: Avascular necrosis of the femoral head in patients on chronic hemodialysis. Trans Am Soc Artif Intern Organs 13:401, 1972.
53. Pinggera, W.F., Popovtzer, M.M.: Uremic osteodystrophy—The therapeutic consequences of effective control of serum phosphorus. JAMA 222:1640, 1972.
54. Ball, J., Johnson, J.W., Hampers, C.L., et al: Many facets of secondary hyperparathyroidism. Arch Intern Med (in press).
55. Wilson, R.E., Bernstein, D.S., Murray, J.E., et al: Effects of parathyroidectomy and kidney transplantation on renal osteodystrophy. Am J Surg 110:384, 1965.

56. Wilson, R.E., Hampers, C.L., Bernstein, D.S., et al: Subtotal para-thyroidectomy in chronic renal failure: Seven year experience in a dialysis-transplant program. Ann Surg 174:640, 1971.
57. Ogg, C.S.: Total parathyroidectomy in treatment of secondary (renal) hyperparathyroidism. Br Med J 4:331, 1967.
58. Bone, J.M., Davison, A.M., Robson, J.S.: Role of dialysate calcium concentration in osteoporosis in patients on hemodialysis. Lancet 1: 1047, 1972.
59. Goldsmith, R.S., Furszyfer, J., Johnson, W.J., et al: Etiology of hyperpara-thyroidism and bone disease during chronic hemodialysis. III. Evaluation of parathyroid suppressibility. J Clin Invest 52:173, 1973.
60. Goldsmith, R.S., Johnson, W.J., Arnaud, C.D.: Value of maintain-ing parathyroid hormone suppressive calcemia in prevention of bone disease and abnormalities in calcium hemeostasis in patients on long-term hemodialysis. Sixth Annual Contractor's Conference, Artificial Kidney-Chronic Uremia Program. Feb. 1973, p 24.
61. Johnson, J.W., Hattner, R.S., Hampers, C.L., et al: Effect of hemo-dialysis on secondary hyperparathyroidism in patients with chronic renal failure. Metabolism 21:18-29, 1972.
62. Alfrey, A.C., Jenkins, D., Groth, C.G., et al: A resolution of hyper-parathyroidism renal osteodystrophy and metastatic calcification after renal homotransplantation. N Engl J Med 279:1349, 1968.
63. Lear, J.: New facts on fluoridation. Saturday Review 52 (9):51–55, 1969.
64. Stare, F.J., Bernstein, D.S., Hampers, C.L., et al: Fluoridation and "new facts." Saturday Review 52(18):57–59, 1969.
65. Merrill, J.P.: *The Treatment of Renal Failure,* ed 2. New York, Grune & Stratton, 1965.

11
Psychological Considerations

Despite progress made in the medical aspects of artificial kidney treatment and the resulting comfort and stability afforded the patient, the
psychological implications of chronic treatment remain burdensome.
Regardless of whether the treatment is performed at home or in the
center, the patient must adjust to the gravity of the situation and change
in life style, and if he is introspective, he must come to grips with
the proposotion of an early death. Regardless of how concrete or
abstract or how disguised these thoughts may be, they usually result
in some behaviorial change. Even the less intellectual patient with
strong denial ability has difficulty in avoiding a reaction to the treatment
which has changed his "normal" existence. The dullest individual will
complain of boredom and the repetitiveness of treatment.

By far the most common psychological manifestation of chronic
dialysis is depression. This is to be expected, of course, and results
from the *real* problems encountered. Once established depression maintains itself at some level throughout the course of treatment, but it
is cyclic in its expression. Certainly the initial confrontation with the
physician and medical staff, the introduction to dialysis and the vicis-
situdes of the early treatment course, result in the most pronounced
and obvious symptoms. At this point, general support is the most
effective therapy, since time usually allows for reactive psychological
adjustments. As the patient begins to feel better medically with the
dialysis treatment and is confronted with other patients in similar situations, some of whom have undergone the therapy successfully, new

hope arises. The time during which severe depression is manifested is variable, depending on the course of the individual patient, but usually subsides after the first few weeks. Depression may worsen if the patient has been unrealistic in what he expects from dialysis and if he does not feel totally "normal" again. In our experience, the use of a psychiatrist during this period is of limited value since the psychiatrist is generally viewed as an outsider with little input or control over the patient's future. The attending physician is best equipped to help the patient and considerable support can also be gained by an enlightened and approachable nursing and technician staff.

Many interpersonal relationships, especially within the immediate family, have a great bearing on the patient's psychological outlook. Family situations which are strained or in which attitudes toward the sick individual change can aggravate the depressive mood. Often the patient is an emotionally strong person who adjusts reasonably well to his illness only to have his problems compounded by the general collapse of his spouse or immediate family. This awesome burden complicates the patient's treatment. An informed social worker or astute and perceptive medical staff can help considerably. Family support is essential and can be of great benefit to the patient. In this instance, in contrast to the treatment of the patient himself, psychiatric consultation may be very helpful. Occasionally family members fear or resent communication with the medical staff and fantasize that this may in some way adversely affect the general outcome. A detached psychiatrist may be quite effective in sympathizing with the family and reconstructing a shattered environment.

It goes without saying that economic considerations surrounding the illness are important stress factors for the patient and the family. The cost of care and sources of payment must be openly discussed early in the encounter with the patient and the family in order to assure a smooth, effective, and nondevasting financial course.

Life psychological patterns are not greatly changed by dialysis. Character traits that have dominated an individual's personality are usually sustained through the early course of renal failure and dialysis, but are exaggerated and characterize the patient's defense reaction to this stressful situation. Patients with great oral needs throughout their lives may find their expression toward their illness one of dietary and fluid indiscretion. It does not take a sophisticated observer to recognize this as a subtle but real suicide attempt. In most instances, the drive is so unconscious enough that it is not recognized by the patient. It may be used to varying degrees. When the fluid balance and dietary indiscretion is of concern to the physician and the medical staff, it may be used as a weapon to rebel against and to frustrate the medical group. Even more commonly, when well meaning family members are concerned and attempt to regulate this aspect of the therapy, dietary intake may be utilized as an infantile, angry slap at the family. It is not uncommon to see a family quarrel, something which heretofore had been vocal and easily expressed, sublimated in the dialysis period and settled (by the patient) through dietary overindulgence.

Although it is difficult to define intentional instances, it is our opinion that the vast majority of dialysis "suicides" occur by this route and are not always appreciated by the family or medical staff. A careful conscious evaluation of this issue should be carried out by the physician on each individual patient. Support, understanding and family counseling may be very important here and can avoid a medical catastrophe. Although the patient generally continues his dietary indiscretion throughout the course of the treatment, it fluctuates in intensity and we feel that it is directly related to stressful situations in the home or in the dialysis unit.

The frightened patient with a high level of anxiety may overcome his anxiety by withdrawal or denial. We encounter a number of patients who remain totally detached from treatment throughout its entire course. Some individuals sleep from the beginning of the dialysis to the end or are seemingly unconcerned. Despite minor crises during the treatment, these individuals may adopt a detached air and on the surface appear to be mature and totally composed. Most of these patients are frightened to death of their illness and are unable to cope directly. This has been their usual pattern in stress situations, although occasionally one sees this characteristic develop in a patient for the first time when confronted with a medical catastrophe of this proportion. In our experience, this type of patient does not respond well to direct confrontation. If the physician is to overcome this attitude he must be warm and understanding. For instance, if the medical staff focuses on one small aspect of the treatment and attempts to totally inform the patient about what is happening and subsequently involves him in this aspect, many of the barriers come down. After an initial period of adjustment, it has been possible to involve such individuals sufficiently so that they can perform dialysis themselves in their home. Some individuals, however, never respond to involvement and any attempt to do so results in further detachment. One must individualize the rapidity and forcefulness with which "involvement" should be approached, but generally this judgment is not difficult.

Role reversal is sometimes necessitated by nature of the dialysis treatment and can cause serious psychological readjustment. This is especially true in inter-relationships involving family members when home dialysis is performed. It also has application, however, to the situation in a dialysis unit, since a certain amount of submissiveness is required in order to have the treatment performed. In the home situation, a previously autonomous family member who is forced to submit may suffer character collapse and be totally ineffective in the day-to-day aspects of his life. If this is compounded by a previously submissive spouse unconsciously taking advantage of the situation in order to have the patient atone for his previous dominance, bizarre consequences can result. Most often neither family member is happy with the reversal of roles and both make some adjustment. Some patients become more autocratic once they develop the obviously submissive role of patient in an attempt to defend their self-image. A patient may become unreasonable, demanding, and almost impossible to relate to during the dialysis procedure. The staff of a dialysis unit is best equipped to handle this reaction since they are less personally involved with the patient and do not present the same magnitude of ego threat. A spouse, on the other hand, may have great difficulty and may need outside help. In this situation both family members need support. This type of psychological interplay between two family members may render them an impossible dialysis team at home, and we have had instances in which the pair has requested return to the center.

Children requiring chronic dialysis may at times become the victim of their parents' previously repressed guilt feelings. When dealing with children, it is particularly important to make certain that parents fully comprehend the problems involved and some time should be spent educating the individuals prior to instituting therapy. Not only must a child be kept free of medical complications, but he must be allowed to return to his previous childhood environment as much as possible. We have seen seemingly intelligent, well-motivated parents actually thwart efforts to rehabilitate their children by what we consider unnecessary overprotectiveness. For example, the parents of a child being encouraged to walk and exercise purchased a wheelchair so that they might spare her physical effort. While most parents realize the importance of education and social rehabilitation, some erroneously believe that a home tutor can replace the benefits expected from the school classroom.

When dialyzing children in a center, we have found it valuable to group children together so that they may share experiences and relationships. Although this plan must be individualized, on the whole it works well.

We initially felt that children would not adjust psychologically to the use of the arteriovenous fistula in that the need for repeated venipuncture would create problems. Much to our surprise, this has not been the case and children learn to tolerate the fistula quite well. As a matter of fact, we believe that as a group children adjust to the venipuncture better than adults.

Sexual function in patients undergoing chronic hemodialysis is variable. In some, no sexual activity at all is desired or engaged in, and in others it is reportedly "normal." This is difficult to predict in the individual patient, but on the whole sexual function as well as libido appears to be limited. The psychological implications of diminished sexual activity, although predictably grave, have not in our experience resulted in major behavioral aberrations. The most important factor here seems to be the spouse's reaction to her partner's loss of libido and her subsequent alteration in behavior. Since the individual patient has low libido, his concern is not over the loss of sex per se, but what effect this is having on the marital partner. Overall, as indicated previously, this has been a minor factor and most patients adjust to this well. We have, however, been aware of some promiscuity on the part of the spouse, but are unable to define the magnitude of the problem.

Several articles have appeared concerning the psychological problems encountered in chronic dialysis patients [1-4]. Although there is some difference of opinion as to the type of appropriate behavior expressed in the individual patients, it seems clear to us that the psychological problems of chronic dialysis patients as a group are not only predictable, but in some ways "normal" given the patients' previous personalities and the facts surrounding their medical illnesses. In other words, psychological adjustment and personality trait exhibition are expected reactions to a real and pressing medical and social situation.

REFERENCES

1. Shea, E.J., Bogden, D.F., Freeman, R.G., et al: Hemodialysis for renal failure: IV. Psychological considerations. Ann Intern Med 62:558, 1965.
2. Abrams, H.S.: The psychiatrist, the treatment of chronic renal failure, and the prolongation of life. I. Am J Psychiatry 124:1351, 1968.
3. Abrams, H.S.: The psychiatrist, the treatment of chronic renal failure and the prolongation of life. II. Am J Psychiatry 126:157, 1969.
4. Wright, R.G., Sand, P., Livingston, G.: Psychological stress during hemodialysis for chronic renal failure. Ann Intern Med 64:611, 1966.

12

Hemodialysis in
the Home Setting

Home dialysis was first introduced in Boston in 1964 [1] and shortly thereafter it was reported in London and Seattle [2.3]. Its development and evolution reflected to some degree the success of maintenance dialysis in general. In the early 1960's, when chronic dialysis was in its infancy, very few hospitals provided such treatment. Those few facilities that did typically had long and often meaningless waiting lists. It was in the spirit of introducing additional facilities for untreated patients that hemodialysis received its initial trial in the home setting. (Figure 1.)

Fortunately, early experience was successful [4,7]. During the initial experience with home dialysis, a physician and nurse were in constant attendance; however, after the first year, their respective roles were gradually curtailed and before long the patient and assistant managed the entire procedure by themselves.

By the mid-1960's, more centers instituted home dialysis training programs. However, it was not until 1967, when the United States Public Health Service funded 12 centers across the country to study the feasibility of home dialysis, that the technique received nationwide application. By 1970, home dialysis was considered by many to be the preferred modality of therapy for chronic renal failure. Some physicians felt so strongly about this that often patients either accepted home hemodialysis or faced death. As a result, some patients were trained for home dialysis who were clearly unsuitable for treatment there. Recognizing the difficulties and the problems encountered in

222

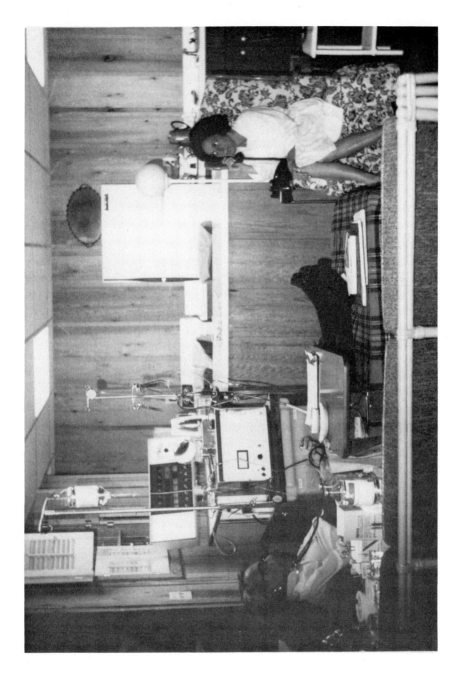

Fig. 1. Home dialysis in an ideal setting.

compelling unsuited patients to perform dialysis in the home, we [8], as well as others, developed out-of-hospital dialysis centers to accomodate this group [9-11]. Requirements for out-of-hospital dialysis units were discussed in Chapter 2.

While much has been said regarding the equipment employed in home dialysis and the dialyzer itself, in overall patient well-being these are less meaningful than stability, support, motivation, and the presence or absence of various contributing medical factors.

Initially access to the circulation was gained by employing first Teflon and then silastic and Teflon arterial and venous cannulae [12,13]. Accordingly, their use and care became an integral part of training. Because cannulae enabled frequent dialyses, home training lessons took place daily and patients were frequently trained and performing treatment at home themselves within 4 weeks. With the advent of the subcutaneous fistula [14], that portion of home training which relates to securing access to the circulation has become somewhat more difficult and prolonged [15,16]. Access to the circulation was discussed in detail in Chapter 3.

Those who use low-flow, low-resistance dialyzers require more hours of dialysis and perhaps more assistant time than those using more efficient dialyzers with blood pumps. However, some have successfully combined dialysis with sleep relying upon monitoring equipment to safeguard them [6,7]. Clearly, the ability to sleep soundly during dialysis without additional risk and without an assistant in attendance represents a strong argument for unattended overnight dialysis. However, not all patients have been able to sleep during dialysis and some have been unwilling to rely solely on monitoring equipment for safety. Accordingly, there has been increasing emphasis on more efficient and shorter dialysis which can be performed during the waking hours. In general, the more vigorous the dialysis, the greater the need for a dialysis assistant.

The initial approach to home dialysis should be one of patient education with familiarization of the system, the procedure, and the personnel involved in the training program. The patient and his assistant should receive a full explanation of all that is involved in their training: the *time* commitments expected of them, the possible consequences —including whatever alterations in life style may be required, the possible medical and technical complications, some assistance in financial planning, and lastly, the exact role each is expected to play in home dialysis and in the training program. In order to properly comprehend what represents to the patient a totally new concept of life, he must be medically and emotionally stable.

When patients have known of their renal failure for some time and have been under competent care during the progression of the disease, it is usually possible to initiate dialysis before medical complications ensue and to prepare the patient emotionally for his dialysis requirements. But it is not uncommon for these patients to deny symptomatology in an effort to defer dialysis. Even the most stable and mature patients remain apprehensive until they actually experience dialysis.

When renal failure develops rapidly over a short period of time or when patients are unaware of the existence of their renal failure, its discovery generally precipitates considerable emotional upheaval. More often than not, patients and families are unable to make rational decisions regarding the acceptability of home dialysis, and when this occurs it is wiser to provide dialysis therapy in a center until the patient and his family can accept thier situations and make necessary adjustments. In such circumstances unit support is most critical. When patients are referred for dialysis late in the course of their disease and medical complications already exist, center dialysis is mandatory until the complications are reversed and the patient is stable and in a reasonable state of health.

During their initial exposure to home training, it has been useful for some patients to meet others who have already experienced home dialysis and who have successfully made necessary adjustments. The sharing of feelings and anxieties has proven quite supportive.

Because considerable professional support is also required for patients undergoing home dialysis training, personnel requirements are substantial and costly. Not only are physicians, nurses, and other direct dialysis personnel necessary, but social service, dietary, and administrative support is required; in many settings, psychiatric or psychologic consultation is beneficial.

The physician responsible for a home dialysis training program serves generally as director and coordinator of staff activities. Aside from assuming routine medical responsibilities, he must determine the frequency and duration of dialysis and the type of equipment to be used, the laboratory studies to be employed and their frequency, the patient's diet and medication, and the time for initiating dialysis. He must also meet with patient and family from time to time and generate a feeling of interest. Therefore, he must be sympathetic and patient as well as attentive and responsive to patients needs, yet firm and resolute when necessary.

Because there is considerable interface between patient and family on one hand and staff on the other, there is more opportunity for personality conflict in a dialysis setting than in most other areas of medicine. The physician director must recognize this and use personnel accordingly. Some patients are openly critical of all staff members, while others express preferences for specific members. It is probably better to acquiesce to a patient's request to provide the nurse he prefers and can relate to for home teaching than to refuse simply to prove a point. Some patients resent the staff because of the continued demand upon their time and the insistence on dietary restraint. The statement "It's easy for you to talk—you don't have to follow these directions" is frequently heard or implied. Other patients project their own problems or inadequacies to the staff. In manipulating these situations the physician must exercise his skills to the greatest degree.

Another problem that may develop because of the continuing relationship between staff and patient is the emotional attachment a staff member may develop toward a patient. This generally interferes with objectivity and may impair the home training program. It is more common with children but does occur with adults. While compassion may often be a virtue, all dialysis patients—and children in particular—are best treated as normally and naturally as possible.

The nurse's role in the home training program is not terribly dissimilar to that of the physician. She serves many of the physician's functions and is the designee of many of his responsibilities. However, she is closer to the patients and in contact with them more.

In order to perform effectively in a home training situation, a nurse must be capable of teaching. However, not all nurses can teach. While one could compile a list of numerous qualities desirable in a nurse, certain traits are particularly important. Maturity, patience, and understanding seem essential to the teaching nurse, as do responsiveness to patients and their problems and ability to relate to others. A teacher must be well versed in his subject matter, and therefore, a nurse teaching dialysis must be totally expert in the use of the artificial kidney and knowledgeable about uremia and its attendant problems. She must understand and be able to explain to patients the rationale of any medications administered. The training environment should convey an air of quiet confidence and professionalism to allay the apprehension and anxiety most patients initially experience.

Aside from teaching responsibilities, the nurse must be aware of the patient's progress and the pertinent information relating to well being. In some programs, nurses are "on call" for home patient problems and accordingly must be familiar with blood pressures, weights, hematocrit levels, and other laboratory studies.

The technician's role in the home training program varies. In some units, the technician may actually participate in patient teaching and share some of the nurse's responsibilities. With the accent on utilization of paramedical personnel, this may tend to increase in the future. In other programs, the technician's role is oriented more toward providing patients with support and technical know-how for equipment maintenance and repair. Still another role of the technician may be in the performance of backup dialysis, when and if necessary.

Social workers are essential to the success of a home dialysis training program. They function primarily in two ways—as information gatherers and evaluators during the initial assessment and as supporters and helpers in the treatment phase. To select the best modality of therapy for a patient, a basic understanding, not only of the patient, but of the family and their interpersonal relationships, must exist. What may superficially appear to be a mature, mutually supportive relationship between two people may actually be considerably less when one looks below the surface. More than any other personnel within a unit, social workers generally possess the expertise to comprehend the realities of the situation. It goes without saying that when family relationships are well understood in advance, problems which may arise are more readily solved.

The social worker's role in resolving problems that occur *during* the treatment stage of home dialysis is less clear. If the problems are temporary, or as often happens, result from misunderstanding or failure to communicate properly, the social worker may effectively restore equanimity. On the other hand, if the problems are due to conflicts between patient and spouse or certain inadequacies in the patient's makeup which relate to the success of home dialysis, we have found the social worker to be no more therapeutically effective than the other members of the team. If the problems are severe enough, home dialysis may have to be abandoned.

The role of the dietician is fairly obvious. However, because patients receiving chronic dialysis have a continuing dietary constraint, more thought and planning must go in to their nutritional requirements than in patients who have short-lived problems or who must make short-term dietary adjustments. To vaguely discuss sodium, potassium, or protein intake and to instruct the patient accordingly is not adequate and will more often than not meet with failure. More properly, a patient's eating habits, as well as his dietary and cultural preferences, need to be considered and a plan formulated which will permit variation and pleasure aside from nutritional requirements. It is probably of value to have the dietician review plans and obtain a nutritional history from patients periodically, determining calories, protein, sodium, and potassium intake. While several groups have reported their experience with modified protein intake in patients undergoing repetitive hemodialysis and others have emphasized the value of high biologic value protein, we have made it our practice *not* to restrict protein in patients once they are being maintained on adequate dialysis and have assumed that with a substantial protein intake sufficient high-biologic value protein is ingested. Furthermore, our experience indicates that patients do better with substantial protein intake and more dialysis than with restricted protein intake and less dialysis. This subject was covered earlier (see Chap. 9).

The administrative responsibility within the home training program relates primarily to financial planning and the purchase of rental equipment and supplies on a continuing basis. Depending upon the size and scope of the program, this role may be fulfilled by a nurse or a technician, or, where programs are of significant size and are a part of larger and more comprehensive renal programs, the role may be filled by a full-time administrator. The original 12 home dialysis training centers funded by the United States Public Health Service in 1967 employed financially capable full-time administrators who developed financial data relative to the cost of home dialysis and researched additional means for the support of ongoing home dialysis programs.

Whereas some years ago it was considered appropriate for a psychiatrist to be directly involved in operating the dialysis unit, there appears to be a growing tendency to call in a psychiatrist only when required, as is done with other specialists. Nevertheless, because of the nature of home dialysis and the stresses it imposes, the need for psychiatric assistance is probably more common than in many other medical situations.

The physical requirements for a home hemodialysis training program are few and simple. First, an attempt should be made to simulate, to the highest degree possible, the home environment. With this in mind, the equipment and supplies dutilized for training should be identical to those employed in the home. The training room should be isolated and separate from the acute or in-center dialysis area and preferably out of the hospital itself. This point has probably not been stressed sufficiently. It may be totally demoralizing for a new patient, about to embark upon home training, to view or become a part of the acute medical problems that arise in maintenance dialysis. The visual impact may severely hinder or even prevent the patient's acceptance of the possibility of resuming a normal life pattern. Examples of home dialysis training areas were shown in Chapter 2.

We have found it helpful to place a telephone in the home training room so that when the patient is no longer nurse dependent, if a problem develops and he requires help, he can call for it by using the phone as he would at home rather than look for a nurse.

Visual aids, particularly the simulated shunt and arteriovenous fistula, have been beneficial in home training. Venipuncture has been troublesome to some patients, and an opportunity to practice and become familiar with handling needles has been very helpful. While more often the patient's assistant assumes the responsibility for venipuncture, some patients accomplish this successfully. In some programs, this has been the procedure of choice, and needles have been designed to enable patients to perform venipuncture more readily.

As experience with home dialysis accumulates and successes as well as failures are re-evaluated, the questions that repeatedly come to mind are: What constitutes an ideal home dialysis candidate? What characteristics and traits predispose toward suuccessful home training? While the answers to these questions have not as yet been clearly or totally defined, certain characteristics important in achieving this goal have been recognized.

First and perhaps most important, is the patient's motivation, including his willingness and ability to participate in his own care. An unwillingness, a lack of desire, or even a reluctance to embark upon home training most often results in an abysmal failure within a short period of time. In our experience, patients who are coerced into attempting home dialysis almost invariably fail and in so doing prove that an error was made from the beginning. However, there are many reasons why patients and their families are concerned about, or question, performing dialysis at home. Sometimes the questions are real and sometimes they are convenient excuses. Apprehension about one's ability to perform successfully, fear of venipuncture, and concern about young children and their contact with dialysis in the home are frequent problems which arise when discussing home dialysis with new patients. These problems are best handled by gentle and sometimes repeated explanation; by exposure to and discussion with other patients; by demonstration of the equipment and patients performing dialysis; and sometimes by gentle introduction to dialysis itself. Many patients respond to this approach and their anxieties are sufficiently alleviated so that they can proceed. However, some patients are resolved against home dialysis and, regardless of the effort expended in explaining the consequences involved, they will not acquiesce. Discretion being the better part of valor, it is best not to even begin home dialysis with these patients.

Patients who are determined to return to their previous roles in society generally do better than patients without immediate goals. Work is perhaps the best example of this, and in general, patients who work do better than patients who do not. Those who are working and those anxious to return to work learn more quickly and accomplish home training more rapidly as a group than those who are unemployed. The dialyzing couple's concern about the training assistant's work time may have the same net effect. We have also found that those who are required to make at least some financial sacrifice by training for home dialysis generally learn more rapidly than those who have no financial stake.

A second vital consideration concerning the success of home dialysis is the patient's stability, his family constellation, and the support the patient receives at home. This is not necessarily easy to evaluate. Often somewhat unstable family situations may seemingly stabilize during a crisis for short periods of time. Patients and their families demonstrate a temporary facade of solidarity, unity, compassion, and understanding for each other even when these emotions never existed previously. Again, the social worker plays a key role in family evaluation. It is important that the staff attempt to understand the family relationships and their currents and counter-currents and anticipate problems that may arise as a result of home dialysis.

It is common for patients to deny the existence of problems during the initial evaluation period. Some problems first surface months later. Many patients have sexual problems resulting from chronic renal failure which they are reluctant to discuss. Sometimes these problems have antedated their renal failure and have required impossible marital adjustments. Occasionally significant communication gaps exist and one marriage partner is unaware of the other's feelings. These feelings may surface and create problems during the months following the onset of dialysis. It becomes very important to fully understand the patient and his family relationship before deciding on the type of care to be offered. To achieve this, sufficient time must be spent with the patient and his family. It is better to defer a decision regarding home dialysis to allow sufficient time for investigation than to make a hasty and sometimes poor judgement.

Once home training begins, several additional stresses may be placed upon the family. The assistant has a new, time-consuming responsibility. An alteration in life style or loss of work may occur with a resultant loss of income. We have observed a number of assistants who have resented the responsibility and burden placed upon them by their sick mates, and a few have expressed a fear of intentionally killing the patient.

In some instances, there has been a reversal in the normal male-female relationship between husband and wife. Men who have had to abandon work as a result of their home dialysis needs and wives who have assumed the role of breadwinner may no longer provide a stable compatible home situation, and we have seen abandonment of home dialysis as well as separation and even divorce result from this. Marriages in which the partners have a sharing relationship have generally resulted in stable home dialysis. Likewise, marriages in which one mate or the other has an obsessive-compulsive personality generally leads to more effective home dialysis. Marriages, however, in which there is a master to servant relationship more often than not result in home dialysis failure.

Some patients, either deliberately or inadvertently, have circumvented some of these problems by engaging medical or paramedical personnel as home dialysis assistants. Of course, a certain degree of affluence is required. We have no real objection to using outside assistants, and even see it as a positive step in certain situations. However, we still feel it is important for the patient and spouse to comprehend home dialysis, know what is required of them, and be able to participate if necessary.

In spite of these problems, we hold that in selected situations home dialysis is the preferred modality of therapy. It is, however, critical that there be a careful and judicious selection mechanism. Unquestionably, it is more convenient and pleasant to receive dialysis at home. Patients are able to set their own schedules according to their needs and alter them as they wish. Some achieve a sense of independence by actively participating in their own care. Those who live long distances from a dialysis center are spared the need to make a burdensome trip repeatedly. Regardless of how pleasant the environment of a dialysis center, it is unlikely to be as comforting to the patient as the cheerfulness and friendliness of his own home. Finally, it is probably less costly to dialyze at home than anywhere else, although when one places a dollar value on assistant time and accounts for some otherwise hidden expenses, the differences in cost between home and center lessen. And there may be no real cost savings when in home dialysis compared to out-of-hospital dialysis centers.

Recently, particularly since the development of out-of-hospital hemodialysis centers, much discussion has centered on the percentage of patients suitable for home dialysis. Our purpose is not to perpetuate the controversy, but rather to attempt simply to place it in some proper perspective. The number of patients suitable for home dialysis may well vary from one population center to another. In a large urban population with a high percentage of socially disadvantaged and economically deprived people, the incidence of suitability for home dialysis is low. On the other hand, in a predominantly rural population—particularly sparsely settled areas—home dialysis seems most applicable. Because nephrologists embroiled in this controversy are dealing with disparate population groups and generally are drawing upon their own experience, disagreement has resulted. Considering our large experience and the population mix that we have been exposed to in Boston and New York, we feel that no more than 25 percent of the people are truly suitable or "good" candidates for home dialysis. We recognize that experience of other workers dealing with different populations has reflected different percentages of patients suitable for home dialysis. Nevertheless, on the basis of our experience we estimate that the national percentage of patients truly suitable for home dialysis is about 33 percent. We emphasize that this is purely an educated estimate.

An additional problem in determining the percentage of patients suitable for home dialysis is patients' therapeutic preferences. We, and others, have encountered patients suitable for home dialysis who prefer to receive treatments in a center.

The results achieved with home dialysis are obviously influenced by the criteria employed in selecting patients and by the patient population encountered. Because criteria and patient mix differ from center to center, one may anticipate some variability in results. It has been amply demonstrated that medically home dialysis is at least the equal of center dialysis [17]. In fact, because of the greater incidence of in-center infection—particularly hepatitis—the home may have a medical advantage. Again, it cannot be overemphasized that this dependends heavily on the population being treated.

As a point of interest, during the last 6 years we have had approximately a 20 percent failure rate in training for home dialysis. Patients who had completed home training required interruption of home dialysis and either returned to the center or requested transplantation as soon as possible. In many cases, devastation reaped upon the family during the home dialysis interval was irrevocable.

REFERENCES

1. Merrill, J.P., Schupak, E., Cameron, E., et al: Hemodialysis in the home. JAMA 190:468, 1964.
2. Shaldon, S.: Proceedings of the Working Conference on Chronic Dialysis. Univ of Washington, Seattle, Dec., 1964, p. 66.
3. Curtis, K., Cole, J.J., Fellows, B.L., et al: Hemodialysis in the home. Trans Am Soc Artif Intern Organs 11:7, 1965.
4. Hampers, C.L., Merrill, J.P., Cameron, E.: Hemodialysis in the home— A family affair. Trans Am Soc Artif Intern Organs 11:3, 1965.
5. Hampers, C.L., Merrill, J.P.: Hemodialysis in the home—Thirteen months experience. Ann Intern Med 64:276, 1966.
6. Eschbach, J.W., Jr., Wilson, W.E., Jr., Peoples, R.W., et al: Unattended overnight home hemodialysis. Trans Am Soc Artif Intern Organs 12: 346, 1966.
7. Baillod, R.A., Comty, C., Ilahi, M., et al: Overnight hemodialysis in the home. Proc Europ Dial Trans Assoc 2:99, 1965.
8. Hampers, C.L., Schupak, E.: Hemodialysis in the home, in Long-Term Hemodialysis, New York, Grune & Stratton, 1967, p. 140.
9. Shapiro, F.L., Messner, R.P., Smith, H.T.: Satellite hemodialysis. Ann Intern Med 69:673, 1968.
10. Billinsky, R.T., Morris, A.J., Klein, H.R.: Satellite Dialysis. JAMA 218:1809, 1971.
11. Neff, M.S., Baez, A., Slifkin, R., et al: Out-patient dialysis. Ann Intern Med (in press).
12. Quinton, W.E., Dillard, D., Scribner, B.H.: Cannulation of blood vessels for prolonged hemodialysis. Trans Am Soc Artif Intern Organs 6:104, 1960.
13. Hegstrom, R.M., Quinton, W.E., Dillard, D.H., et al: One year's experience with the use of indwelling Teflon cannulas and bypass. Trans Am Soc Artif Intern Organs 7:47, 1961.
14. Brescia, M.J., Cimino, J.E., Appel, K., et al: Chronic hemodialysis using venipuncture and a surgically created arteriovenous fistula. N Engl J Med 275:1089, 1966.
15. Schupak, E., Singer, A., Casey, J.D.: Home hemodialysis with subcutaneous arteriovenous fistula. JAMA 210:4, 1969.
16. Shaldon, S., McKay, S.: Use of internal arteriovenous fistula in home hemodialysis. Br Med J 4:671, 1968.
17. Gross, J.D., Keane, W.F., McDonald, A.K.: Survival and rehabilitation of patients on home hemodialysis: Five years experience. Division of Prof. & Tech Devel, Regional Medical Programs Service. Health Services; Mental Health Administration, Rockville, Md, 1972.

Index

3 a
4 b
5 c
6 d
7 e
8 f
9 g
0 h
1 i
8 2 j